Nurse Call

"WHEN I GROW UP I'M GOING TO BE A NURSE"

Penelope Frances

Melbourne Australia

Penelope Frances c/- Intertype Publishing
Unit 45, 125 Highbury Road
BURWOOD VIC 3125
www.intertype.com.au

Book Layout ©2020 by Intertype

Ordering Information:
Quantity sales. Special discounts are available on quantity purchases by corporations, associations, and others. For details, contact the "Special Sales Department" at the address above.

Nurse Call / Penelope Frances —1st ed.
ISBN 978-0-6487977-0-8

Contents

If you require support for any issues raised, then please contact

Lifeline: ph. 131114
www.lifeline.org.au
1800respect (domestic and family violence/ sexual assault):
www.1800respect.org.au
Sands (miscarriage, stillbirth loss): ph. 1300 072 637
www.sands.org.au

Dedication
To my dear children (My Three Amigos)

Gavin: When you put your first finger up for "Just one more?" cuddle before I went to work.

Michael: When you would block the front door with your little arms and legs in the hope, I would not leave for work but stay home with you.

Amanda: When you would hide my car keys in your toy box, then grab my leg in tears as I headed off to work with my spare set.

My Mum: Who sadly passed during the writing of this book. I hope I made you proud

My Brother, John: I never got to say goodbye to you. This is for you

My Grandchildren (both current and future): Never give up on your dreams!

My Family: May we always appreciate how lucky we are to have each other and enjoy each moment spent together.

Foreword

"When I grow up, I am going to be a nurse" At the tender age of 9 there were no "ifs or buts". This is a story of my amazing journey. As a young girl, I grew up on a farm as a tomboy, eating dirt and nurturing animals. My path to becoming a fully-fledged nurse, fraught with obstacles. I share my hardships and joys with you. I have retraced my experiences with some unforgettable characters. These stories will make you laugh, cry and appreciate how incredibly precious life is. I wrote this book over eight years. I am now teaching beautiful, student nurses. Let us hope they make a positive difference every single day. If this book helps just one person, I consider its production well worthwhile! I hope you enjoy reading this as much as I enjoyed writing it – Penelope Frances.

Acknowledgement

To my dear friend Melissa Walsh for her friendship since our school days and for editing "Nurse Call". You have been a close confidant and I am lucky to have you in my life. I thank you for your love, encouragement and support. May our friendship continue well into our twilight years

Introduction

"The grey nurse," just the mere mention of these three words were enough to make your hairs stand on end for those who worked at a certain well-known hospital in the northern suburbs. Many stories had circulated and had been told and retold by staff within the hospital. The "grey nurse" was seen on many occasions by staff as she walked the dimly lit passageways of the hospital at night.

She appeared, clad in the original nurse uniform, worn in the early 1900s, calmly attending to her duties, well beyond her living years. Her presence was reported by not only medical/nursing staff but also by her beloved patients. Her work would happen when the sun went down. She would tirelessly travel the hospital, quietly assisting a needy patient, often giving a blanket, tucking them in, or lending a helping hand if required. Just when it was thought she may finally have moved on she would appear yet again to another unsuspecting person and set tongues wagging. I believe we experienced a visit from this angel of the night on a ward I was nursing on.

It was the year 1988 and it was a busy night. My co-worker and I had finally settled down at the nurses' desk to tally up our fluid balance charts for the day. This involved calculating the total amount of fluid a patient had received in a full 24 hour period, then subtracting the total amount of fluid that patient had excreted to see if the patient was in a positive or negative balance regarding fluids (it ideally should be completed by midnight 24:00). It was well after, as it had taken a long time to settle our patients tonight. The majority were post-operative, which meant we had dressings to do on their wounds, make them pain-free by administering their analgesics, and a lot were on intravenous antibiotics. Finally, we managed to sit down. I made a cup of steaming Earl Grey tea for Annie and I made a strong Nescafe. As we sipped on our drinks, we attempted to get our paperwork done. It was unusually quiet; there was not a moan, or noise heard. Outside, the cold wind was howling as it whipped between the buildings and I paused for a second to listen. I hated this part of the shift. Math was not my favourite pastime and all the figures I seemed to lose track of, as I deftly entered them into my calculator at lightning pace speed. Bother! I had to go back and repeat this to make sure I had got it right. With a yawn, I completed this task, whilst sipping on my caffeine-loaded beverage. Thank god for coffee! Without it … I'm sure I'd be nodding off into dreamland about now!

Then, I glanced over at Annie, as we heard an elderly voice call us. "Hello … who's there?" I jumped up, in the direction of Mrs Brown's room. She was a sweet, gentle lady who had been inflicted with ovarian cancer. She was in the end stage of her awful disease and was unable to walk anymore. I thought she may need toileting, as her cancerous tumours had spread invading her bladder and it wasn't uncommon that she would wake frequently bursting for a wee.

As I entered her room, which she shared with three others, I glanced to the left side, where her bed was occupied. The night lights glowed underneath all beds, from the walls but it took me just a few seconds for my eyes to adjust to make out objects in the semi-darkness. I pulled my torch out of my pocket and shone it along the floor, moving quietly in her direction but I bumped her chair which was obstructing my access to her bed. That's strange I thought. I was very particular that at the beginning of my shifts I would clear the room from clutter, pushing back all chairs to leave a clear pathway to my patients, particularly at night, as the lighting was poor. I shone my little torch upwards and saw Mrs Brown laying back in the chair which was reclined. The cot side on my side was down and Mrs Brown looked up at me and smiled saying, "It was lovely for that nurse to get me out of bed and set me up in my chair but I have had quite enough now and I think I will try to get some sleep. Thank you, dear." I must have had a puzzled look on my face, as I glanced behind me to find Annie looking over, just as astonished. I looked back at Mrs Brown. "Mrs Brown, who got you out of bed? What did she look like?" Mrs Brown replied, "It was a nurse, I think she was a nun, dressed in grey. I didn't get her name. But she was a kind lady. She didn't say much. Now get me back into bed please, if you have a moment." The bed had been folded back and as neat as a pin. Not a wrinkle could be seen, unlike the beautiful deep wrinkles etched deeply in its occupant's face. I put Mrs Brown on a commode chair and wheeled her off to the toilet, before tucking her in soundly, yet again for the night.

As I locked her cot side into place once more, I looked at Mrs Brown's sleepy face and found comfort in the fact that she appeared more relaxed than I'd seen her for a long time. Her eyes were now closed but you couldn't mistake the smile that was planted on her face as she fell asleep. I rubbed her on the hand and said, "Goodnight." Maybe Mrs Brown had a visit of a ghostly kind that evening? But I knew then, if the grey nurse was still looking over us then there was nothing to fear … she did no harm. Perhaps to the contrary. Mrs Brown slept through the night, without stirring and did not wake once with the discomfort of her annoying bladder.

If I were to encounter the grey nurse wandering our passages now, I'd personally thank her for giving dear Mrs Brown one night of complete rest … and I'd want to know more about this remarkable lady and her life. Why did her devotion to nursing continue well beyond her living years?

CHAPTER 1

A Nurse In The Making

Unlike most of my friends at school, I always knew what I wanted to do when I left college. I attended a Catholic all-girls' school. We were nick-named by surrounding colleges the "brown cows" due to our uniform that consisted of a tunic, tie, hat and gloves. From the age of five, where I grew up on a wheat and sheep property in the Western District of Victoria, I'd roam the paddocks in the tractor or on foot, always looking for an adventure. I was not into the tea sets and dolls that my older sister enjoyed. She would help mum indoors, cook and clean whilst I was outside happily making mud pies, helping dad round up sheep or lying in the wheat fields, just gazing up at the clouds, floating, across the sky, making out their shapes and daydreaming. I'd hear in the distance mum calling me in for supper. I'd jump up, skipping to the farmhouse, sponged in dirt from my head to my toes. I was a tomboy, unlike my sister who had the graces and ladylike airs of a princess. I'd be marched into the bathroom and the bath would be run with ice-cold water while mum fetched the hot water, which had boiled, on the fire stove in the kitchen. The water would be lukewarm but after I'd had my bath it was cold and dirty black but my blonde hair, golden again.

My favourite pastime and memories of my childhood on our farm were the animals. I adored them … when baby calves were born, I'd be there to help deliver them if they were stuck. I remember rearing them by hand when their mothers died from the birth. Cows have the biggest, most loving eyes and the calves would suck at their bottle so hard, the milk would gush into their mouths quickly until every drop was savoured and gone. I enjoyed being their adopted mother as they followed me around everywhere. As a child, the animals received most of my attention and I clearly remember mum commenting that I had such a big heart; one day I would kill something with so much love. I loved animals with all my heart.

At the tender age of five, I knew I wanted to be a nurse when I grew up. I never even considered any other career. At the age of eight, my parents separated, and my mum brought us to Melbourne. The saying, "You can take the girl out of the country – but not the country out of the girl," is so true. I feel at peace, relaxed and at home still, only when I am in the wide-open spaces of the country. To this day, I hope one day to return to the country life to live.

I don't wish to bore you with a prolonged version of my childhood, but I wanted to share with you a brief look at my background as I believe by going back to my roots, I can understand why I wanted to be a nurse.

On the farm, I saw the cycle of life in its purest form. I experienced birth, death, sickness, injury, cruelty and disease in many forms. Animals taught me so much. And I loved every creature equally. They could not tell me if they were sick, or in pain. I just knew, intuitively when something was wrong. I often nursed them back to health with the most basic requirements for life: warmth, food and water but mostly love and compassion. I took the time to get to know each animal's needs. Maybe this is why I specialized in Paediatric nursing? Children can't always tell you in words what is wrong with them. It's only by knowing children's natures and by observing their body language that you can pick up on what's wrong with a child, only then can you treat them appropriately. Both children and animals are innocent and vulnerable and need protecting but everyone at some stage of their lives needs someone to help them. No matter how strong, or healthy, or proud, or rich, every single one of us has our turn to be humbled.

I nurse by my instincts and intuition … on many occasions I've drawn on these, as they tell me something's wrong and I act on this immediately. My instinct … has never let me down. It allows me to act earlier, rather than later and I believe this is the most reliable tool I use in nursing. I developed this invaluable tool as a child and unlike sight, smell, taste, touch and hearing, it can never be taken away from me. It will never deteriorate. It's my sixth sense and is the most precious sense I own. I am so grateful that I had the opportunity to be raised in the country as it's there that I started my nurse training.

I failed English by one mark in my VCE year! When I received my results via post, I was shaking in anticipation when I opened my letter. I couldn't believe what I was reading. 49% … This meant I'd failed the whole year. Okay, I enjoyed socializing! I hadn't studied for hours each night! Half an hour usually sufficed to complete the allocated work. Yes, I crammed to study the night before an exam! What was this though? I'd failed?

I was a bright girl, who usually took everything in, the first time. For sure, I was different from my older sister, next in line, who studiously went over all her work that day, every night, for hours on end. But did I deserve this? No way! Nevertheless, there was nothing I could do about it now. The results were there on paper, glaring back up at me in the black print. An unmistakable fail!

My family tiptoed around me that day and tried to console me as best they knew how. But this result meant I couldn't commence my nursing training unless I repeated my VCE year. Bother, there was no way I could go back to the same school and face those teachers another year; it would surely kill me! So, I discussed my options with mum and I decided to repeat the year in a new environment, boarding school. There was an establishment run by the nuns on the outskirts of Ballarat.

There I would be with girls from all over Victoria and I adored Ballarat. It was not far from my birthplace and the place where I grew up! Mum agreed that it was a good idea and after the summer holidays at home, I commenced at this catholic school and had an amazing year, packed with adventure, new friends and to top it off, at the end of this amazing experience I achieved the successful completion of my Year 12. This victory meant that finally, I could achieve my dream of training at my chosen hospital that was in the city of Melbourne. I couldn't have been happier! On February 11th, 1983, I was to start my formal nursing training. I never realized that day was the beginning of lifelong devotion, not just a career, but also much more than that. At the age of nearly 18, I was a young, naïve woman who had so much to learn. I thought I knew it all. I had no idea! Probably just as well.

Recently I had a student nurse who came to our hospital for placement. She had just turned seventeen and reminded me a lot of myself when I first started. This day she looked at me and said, "You have to mature very quickly when you become a nurse, don't you?" I looked at her and replied, "Yes, you do." I wanted to protect her in a way from the harsh realities that she would come across but knew she would need to experience things and deal with them in her way, as we all need to. She was just one of a small group of students who were a pleasure to teach and eager to learn. On their last day, a group of four of them approached me on my own and thanked me for what I did for them. I was very touched by this gesture and had a tear in my eye as I said to them that if they needed someone to talk to, I was always here for them. They gave me a big hug and that was it. I hate goodbyes to this day. There are many goodbyes in nursing. I find these so sad, but they are balanced out, with many hellos as well. I have befriended people from all walks of life, all cultures, all different socio-economic backgrounds but none of these things alter the way I feel and care about any individual. They are all my brothers and sisters and family and I treat them as such. I laugh with them and I cry with them as I am one of them.

In the classroom, I'd breezed through the classes, passed all my tests but how was I going to deal with injecting real patients, not oranges, which we had practised our injections on tirelessly before. I felt sick with worry as I headed to our cafeteria to have some breakfast before work, not that I felt much like eating but I thought it may help me from feeling sick on the job.

We were given a tour of our ward, met our charge nurse and were promptly assigned to a mentor nurse for the day. The handover was so quick. I hardly had time to put pen to paper before we were onto the second patient. They may as well have been talking another language as I struggled to keep up and by the end of it, my head was spinning, my spelling was atrocious and even I couldn't understand what I'd scrawled on my handover sheet.

My mentor was a nurse in her mid-twenties, whom I followed in her every footstep that day. I was her shadow she couldn't shake. She had a friendly, warm disposition and the patients all smiled when she first came into their rooms that day, all except for one, Mr Collier. As we approached Mr Collier to greet him, I noticed a pungent, strong smell of stale urine that took my breath away. Sam my mentor approached him, gently touching his arm. "Good morning Mr Collier. How was your night?" He glared at her through his steel-blue eyes and snapped, "What is it to you?" Sam replied, "Breakfast will be here soon. How about we give you a nice hot shower, so you are all ready for the day." She glanced over at me as she pulled his blankets back and deftly whipped a pair of disposable gloves from a box on the bedside table and motioned me to do the same. I clumsily put a pair of gloves on and attempted to assist Sam in getting this man out of bed. As she took the top end, I took his legs and we swung him into a sitting position. While my head was down, I felt a large whack aimed at the side of my head that caught me completely off guard. I tried to put my head up as the whole room was spinning but alas, not to be. Mr Collier grabbed me in a headlock and my head was firmly planted under his odorous armpit. I was completely helpless and pinned down by his big hairy arm. But not his prisoner for long, within seconds I felt his grip release and as I came up quickly for air. I noticed Sam had saved me from Mr Collier's clutches. She had a bemused look on her face as she assisted me upright and attempted to straighten my hat, hair and dress in one sweep. I learned quickly to keep at arms' length from Mr Collier to prevent this from ever happening again. Yet I learned to attend to all his nursing care needs meticulously too, always ensuring I could quickly escape his clutches if the need arose again. This was the start of the developing observation, assessment and evaluation skills that are the essence of every nurse.

My nursing training was at a large Catholic hospital in Melbourne. It was only natural that I chose to train there as I was baptised and raised a catholic. I had attended mass every Sunday with my family. I was used to nuns' discipline and curfews. We had to be home by 10:00 pm or nurses' home doors were locked. It was then necessary to come in through the hospital's underground route, a journey that was like a rabbit warren with the main tunnel that would take you past the mortuary. I shivered when I walked past that cold white door, a place I would soon get to know much better.

What happens to us when we die? There is much published about the 'afterlife' and to this day, I am very intrigued by the number of varied but special experiences I have had. I have been privileged enough to be there, at the moment of a persons' death on many occasions. I do know that a 'journey' occurs as the soul leaves the body. I have witnessed many wonderful moments that I will forever cherish and as a nurse, I can never under-estimate the importance of our role in providing comfort, care and company at this time.

I had a dear nursing colleague whom I visited in ICU the day before she died. Mary was being kept alive by medical technology, equipment and medications. She was 'unconscious' or so her nurse, caring for her this day, advised us. I went and sat on a chair next to her and picked up her limp hand and held it in mine. As I began to chat with her, I felt her squeeze my hand, not once, but many times. I knew beyond a doubt that this beautiful lady was letting me know she was pleased I was there for her. In the few months before this, I had visited her in hospital, and she was off having x-rays, so I had missed seeing her but left a gift on her bedside table. A week later I came home from work and found a card sitting on my doorstep with a picture of a cat on the front and inside the card were the words, "You always know I've visited by the gift I leave." Inside the card, the cat had a dead mouse on a doorstep. Mary loved cats and her card let me know that she had appreciated my visit and a small gift. I went home after seeing Mary in ICU and knew I would not see her again. The next morning, she died. I still have the card she left me.

CHAPTER 2

Making A Difference

My first death as a student nurse, was in coronary care. I was on student placement for two weeks in this unit and this evening I was sitting at the desk, watching the cardiac monitor on which all the inpatients were wired up to, so their ECG was clearly visible in the nurses' station. I was becoming vaguely familiar with how to read an 'ECG' (electrocardiogram) when suddenly a gentleman's trace on the screen showed his heart rate slowing. It was normally around 60 beats per minute and it rapidly dropped to 28 beats per minute and then the trace flat-lined. I jumped to my feet as the monitor pierced my ears with its alarm. The senior nurse on duty, who was standing behind me discussing a patient's condition with a cardiologist, darted a quick look at the screen, then ran quickly to the patient's room with the doctor closely in tow. I followed behind and upon entering the room I saw Brian, the patient semi-propped on his pillow, in the same position he had been watching television just seconds before. He had closed his eyes and was becoming paler by the second.

Brian had cardiomyopathy and his heart was very weak and other than a new heart, he had a very limited chance of living a long life without an 'organ donation'. He was 'NFR' – not for resuscitation. I felt helpless, as a student nurse, it was difficult to just stand by and watch. But he was gone. At the tender, youthful age of twenty-eight years he was taken and there was nothing more that could be done. I watched the nurse in charge approach this young man and touch him gently on the cheek as if to say goodbye and I noticed a teardrop in the corner of her eye as she turned to the doctor and spoke to him of notifying family. The doctor nodded to her as she left the room and he listened intently to Brian's silent chest, ensuring all signs of life had ceased. I stood at the door for another minute watching as if suddenly Brian would just open his eyes and maybe it was just a bad dream. But I was brought back to reality by a gentle touch on my shoulder and the nurse in charge prompted me to realise that my services were required as I was asked to get a water bowl, towel and washers to assist in giving Brian his last sponge before his family arrived.

I prepared the bowl of warm water, fetched the towels and washers and with arms laden, my hands holding onto the round green bowl, I headed towards Brian's room. There was already a sign on the door, 'DO NOT ENTER'. I knocked, feeling a bit silly. What was I expecting? Brian to answer? Nothing! I struggled with the door handle and entered Brian's room without spilling a drop. It was eerily quiet as I cautiously made my way to the bedside table. Somehow, Brian was now lying flat with his head gently elevated on only one pillow. I felt uneasy, alone with Brian's body. This uneasiness grew with each passing moment. I had never seen a dead person before, yet here I was, alone in a room with one. I heard my heartbeat loudly in my ears as I got ready to flee the room. I heard the door click and I jumped just as Josie entered the room. Phew ... I was so relieved it was her! Josie was a middle-aged nurse who had a thick mop of sparkling grey hair that always looked neat as a pin. She was just coming on for the night shift and was popping in to check on Brian before his relatives arrived. She smiled that familiar smile. I was so relieved to see her! "Hello, dear.

What are you still doing here? Don't tell me they left you here alone? Off you go sweetheart. Time for you to knock off. I will finish this up." With a grateful smile, I told Josie that I would like to stay and help with Brian. I explained to her that he was my first patient who had passed. Josie understood and I'm sure she noticed my trembling hands as she replied, "Okay then."

We pulled the blinds down and washed Brian from top to toe. We spoke to him as if he could hear us. I'm sure he was listening from somewhere. We explained what we were doing and kept him modestly covered, only exposing where we washed. We dried, powdered, even put aftershave on him. Then changed his bed with crisp white starched sheets. He glowed with cleanliness, whilst all the time he appeared to be sleeping peacefully. Brian looked amazing when we accompanied his mother into the room. We had found a beautiful red rose that we had gently laid on his pillow. I asked his mum if she would like me to stay but as she stroked Brian's head, with tears leaking from her eyes, she asked to spend some time alone with him. My heart was heavy as I walked out of Brian's room, like a stone had lodged and was stuck there and I wondered if this heaviness would ever lift. I found Josie preparing tea in an elegant gold trimmed teapot, with a matching cup and saucer. She went to the fridge and scrounged around until she found some white sandwich triangles with egg and lettuce, gherkin and cheese. After it was beautifully laid out on the silver serving tray, she looked me in the eye and said, "There you go love, this is for Brian's mum." I took the tray and walked back to the room, knocking before I entered and saw Brian's mum sitting on the chair with her head resting gently on her son's chest. She had not heard me enter, so I started pouring the steaming hot tea into the cup and walked to the opposite side of the bed. Her head lifted and I offered her the tea. Her red rimmed eyes closed as she sipped, trying to find comfort in the tea's warmth. She looked at me as I offered her a sandwich and she thanked me. Scoffing down the sandwiches she appeared more at ease and I sat with her for a while. She shared with me the wonderful memories she had with her precious son. She had lost her husband a few years earlier and Brian was her only child.

I felt so humbled to be able to share this precious time with Brian's mum and to cry and laugh and just be there for her. I now knew why I had become a nurse. To be there for people at their lowest, saddest, sickest, most vulnerable moments. Everyone who is born into this world will one day die. Some will have short lives, like Brian and some live long lives. Everyone at that moment of death will pass over into another realm. To be there for someone at this special, once in a lifetime moment, to comfort them and make that transition easier for them is an absolute privilege. God giveth life … and only God can taketh away. We may not know when, or how or even why. One thing I do know is the peace and knowledge that there is something wonderful to behold in the life after and beyond our world.

Once Brian's mother had left; Josie and I had the final duty of preparing his body for the mortuary. Back in the early 1980's, much to my distaste, all orifices were packed with cotton wool, then the body was wrapped in a large, thick, plastic black sheeting. The end above the head was secured with thin string or material tape, to which a yellow tag identifying the body was attached. The plastic was then tightly gathered at the end of the feet and secured again with string and another ID tag. When this procedure was completed, Josie said, "There you go love, that's how you go off … like a big bonbon." To this day I will never forget looking at what we had done and thinking, "Oh dear, that's exactly what it looks like!"

CHAPTER 3

Fit For A King

Death does not come easy for some … thankfully though, more dignity I felt was shown, as the years went on and a time came when we were no longer required to use cotton wool to prepare them for their journey. People were washed then placed in their best pyjamas or such instead of the old hospital gowns. As a student, I was horrified by the use of cotton wool! The black plastic was also discarded, thank Goodness! People are now lying comfortably in a bed to await the gentlemen or ladies from the funeral home to arrive. In some nursing homes the departed are escorted through the front door, not out the back door, as they originally arrived, but respectfully through the front door, So this is the manner also in which they should finally leave the establishment. Very dignified indeed! Many changes for the better have eventuated over the years to benefit our dearly departed.

Peter was a homeless gentleman who occupied our hospital bed on many occasions. I was a registered nurse just qualified when I first met this cheery and intriguing character. He and I had a special bond and from the first time I met him, something just clicked, and we became 'close buddies' … in a work/patient sense. Peter always came in smelling of alcohol, his clothes torn and filthy, hanging off his emaciated frame like a wet, worn coat hanger. His hair would be matted, his beard long and ratty, his stomach protruding over his tracksuit pants band like a tear drop shaped, water filled balloon – all ready to pop.

Without exception, no matter how frail and sickly he was on admission, he would see me walk in on my shift and beam the biggest smile at me, flashing the whitest teeth. His face was tinged in yellow due to his liver failure, a by-product of his fondness of alcohol.

I would always ensure he was thoroughly clean, although it was as if the dirt was never ending when I assisted him with his initial shower. I'd soak his feet in bowls of soapy water to try and budge the ingrained filth that coated his soles of his feet. I scrubbed them until they were almost pink again. I would then set him up at the sink with the razor and soap, where we would commence the arduous process of 'shaving'. He would only shave when he came to hospital, but I would refer to this as a 'shear' on Peter. After a few nicks and placing tissues on these to stem the bleeding, he would emerge from the bathroom a 'different' man. In a matter of half an hour he would change identity. I would always track down some hospital men's flannel, striped PJs which he would slip into. I'm sure every visit he would look and more importantly, feel like a new man.

It is true; we cannot have favorite patients. Nurses should have the quality to treat all equally, regardless of age, race, religion, culture, socio-economic situation and gender. I pride myself with this quality and I genuinely believe that to be void of all prejudice and have a deep compassion for all people from different walks of life is the key ingredient for nursing.

Peter would sit up in his green striped hospital pyjamas and look out over the city, like a king perusing his kingdom. He was usually always allocated to the same single room each visit, which afforded him spectacular views across to the horizon. He particularly enjoyed the lights shining at night and was always reluctant to close his mini venetians.

He loved football and his team was St Kilda. He had a small TV dangling from the wall, which he could just relax in bed and watch his team play on a Saturday. The only thing he loved more than his footy was his mealtimes.

The catering staff would place his tray on his over bed trolley, and he would sit up straight and tall in bed. Then he would remove the covers of each plate and bowl and savour the sight and smell of his meal thoroughly, before he would devour every morsel and chew each mouthful as if it were his last. You would think, being homeless he would lack good table etiquette. To the contrary, he was very adept at using all cutlery and held it with great finesse. He would never rush his meals either; in fact, he would take twice as long to finish his meal as anyone else. He did not like to be rushed. Mealtime was sacred!

It had been a few months since Peter had been admitted. This was unusual and I wondered to myself how he was doing. Then I arrived to work one day and was told Peter would be transferred to the ward from casualty, as we had no beds available in the past two days. In the past few days he had been kept in casualty awaiting a bed.

On my return I found Peter in his usual room, very dishevelled as usual but looking particularly yellow this time. Peter had end stage liver failure from liver cirrhosis – ethanol abuse. Alcohol was the poison that Peter could not live without. It was common knowledge that we would treat Peter's liver failure until he would eventually succumb to the disease. In the case of death, Peter had made it clear that he wanted to go, without a fuss. He was made 'Not for Resuscitation' (NFR) by the covering liver Registrar upon discussing the options with Peter and listening to Peter's wishes.

Peter greeted me as he looked up with the most wonderful smile. Everything lit up on his face, like a beacon in the night. I was shocked by Peter's sunken eyes and thin face, even visible beneath his woolly beard. He said, "Hi, how are you my dear girl? Have you been keeping well my dear?". Here, this wonderful sweet-hearted man was asking me how I was, when it was blatantly obvious, he was desperately unwell. I could not help but smile back! I told him I was great as I ran over to check his intravenous line to ensure he was getting the required fluids he desperately needed. His lips were dry, cracked and bleeding like the parched soil in a desert that had cracked wide open from lack of moisture. I hurried over to the supplies draw and immediately pulled out the lip balm which I gently patted on his lips with a gloved finger. Now, he was up to date with all his prescribed medication. "Good!", I thought as I flicked through his drug chart and doctor's orders. "Time for a wash Peter". "That would be lovely, I could do with a bit of a spruce up you know!", he replied. Peter was too weak today to tolerate a shower, so he would need a sponge in bed. After this, he looked and felt a bit better. I then shaved him and scrubbed his teeth until they were white and glistening in his mouth like the pearl jewels of the Nile! He sighed and smiled at me, sinking deeper into his warm comfy bed. I fetched him a warm blanket from the blanket warmer to wrap around his freezing cold body and he was snug again in his favorite hospital PJs. I thought he was about to have a well-deserved sleep but low and behold, dinner was served. Peter's eyes flicked open at the sound of the dinner trolley rattling along outside his room and I saw him drag himself up to a sitting position like a lion, ready to pounce on his prey. He was almost drooling from one corner of his mouth as the food arrived in front of him.

As I watched on, I noticed he was too frail to remove the covers from his food, so I sat down next to him and said, "Peter, how about I give you a hand with this meal fit for a King?" He just smiled and nodded as I placed his serviette over his top and started feeding him. He took his time, savouring and chewing each mouthful as if it were his last. He looked like the cat that just swallowed the cream. When he was done, the plate was clean. I joked with him about 'not even leaving enough scraps on it for the kitchen staff to clean'. I noticed he was resting back on his pillow now just gazing intently at me. He smiled and said, "Now I am ready to die". I saw his eyes glaze over, I noticed him sigh, then nothing. He was gone! I reached over and closed his eyes for the very last time. I knew he had gone to a better place. I knew he had died comfortably and with dignity. He had a smile still apparent on his peaceful, gentle face. He had lived as a pauper … but my friend Peter, he had died as a King.

CHAPTER 4

What A Relief

Nursing in the mid 1980's was very different than today. There was no such thing as nurse ratios. You just took whatever allocation you were given and organised your shift accordingly. After lunch each day was pan room duty, where we would be required to check each bottle and pan to ensure they were gleaming and clean. This room was spotless and always meticulously kept.

Our training was strict; if we didn't perform a procedure correctly, follow the process that was ingrained into our minds, we were brought down then and there by our clinicians, often in the presence of the patient who would grimace at the manner in which we were spoken to. I would just blush with sheer embarrassment and apologise to the patient who often I felt, shared our humiliation as much as we did.

I am a big advocate for professionalism. To me, throughout my practise, I always reflect on these early training years and I learnt to never reprimand any colleague in the presence of other patients, nor other staff, nor visitors. I learned a valuable lesson about respect. I carry this message through, in my current clinical facilitator role. I would never ask the student nurses I facilitate, nor anybody for that matter, to perform a task in which I myself was not willing to roll up my sleeves and do.

There are many instances where a student nurse has commented to me about 'being left with all the menial tasks' I ask them what they mean by 'menial'. The reply is often that because they are 'students' they are left to do 'all the showers' or 'all the vital signs'. I explain to them that these so-called 'menial' jobs are as vitally important as the jobs they would prefer to be doing. One of these jobs they often enjoy learning is administering medication. My question here is, how can you administer medications unless the vital signs are taken, recorded and known by the nurse administering medication? For example, when a person is showered, so much vital information is gained by the nurse performing this task. Assessments during this shower include – how much assistance do they need to shower properly? Can they wash all parts of their body thoroughly or do you need to assist them with certain tasks? Such as hair washing, or ensuring they can stand safely, to wash their private areas or any folds in their skin. Can they dry themselves thoroughly, ensuring all areas and skin are clean and dry, with no rashes, breaks or any redness? These issues need to be attended to immediately by evaluation, reporting to a superior, and putting a care plan in place, in collaboration with other colleagues. Treating issues promptly and instigating correct care is often the key to halting any deterioration in the patient's condition.

A big problem that can occur with nursing, is when all of a client's care needs are performed, without encouraging and waiting to see what the client can achieve for themselves . This may reach the point where the patient has all of their independence taken away from them. They can quickly become reliant on this help and expect everything to be done for them. It is crucial that we, as nurses, maintain a patient's independence by encouraging them to do as much as possible. Certainly to 'assist' them with activities they are struggling with. Importantly, observe closely and educate patients on caring and understanding their limitations and how they can better overcome them. This helps clients with any frustrations. If we are always there offering our support, this will encourage them to feel more independent, confident and positive about their condition and how to maintain their most optimal health, whilst having all their care needs met.

I strongly encourage all nursing students to develop a close rapport with their clients by being 'present' when they are with them. Listening carefully, making good eye contact and spending quality time with each individual, helps us to meet all their needs as we understand and respond to this client appropriately and respectfully.

Look at a client who is constantly pressing their nurse buzzer for what might appear to be trivial things. If you take the time to go in and listen to them, you may find that they may feel quite scared or lonely. They may indeed have something that is easily remedied. Always take precious time out of your busy day to spend with this client and really listen to them.

A good example of this, is in the following story of a man who was in a great deal of pain. I looked up to find two of my nursing students walking quickly towards me. They asked me if I could see a gentleman as he was complaining of persistent pain. One of these students had a very concerned look on her face so I immediately asked the students to lead the way. As I approached this man's room, I could hear him cursing away to himself. Most of the words he muttered were incomprehensible but in between these I could hear the words 'stupid' and 'staff' and 'left to die'.

This gentleman was facing away from the door, as he lay askew on the messy bed, his sheets lay tousled and strewn, dragging on the floor. I knocked quietly on the door and entered, asking the students to wait for me outside, so as I could beckon them in if permission from this man was sought and gained.

Mr Finch turned his top half toward the door to check who was there. I had briefly met Mr Finch the day prior to this, to supervise a student with performing a blood glucose level (BGL) reading. "May I come in Mr Finch?" I asked and he replied quite gruffly with an aggravated, "Come in!", he proceeded to look me in the eyes saying, "I've had enough of this place! I am going to walk out of here soon. No-one does anything for me. I have had this pain in my leg all day and no one has even bothered to take the time to help me!". He had a look of sheer exasperation on his face and he spoke loudly, his face became redder as he appeared to become even angrier.

I calmly asked Mr Finch if he minded if I looked at his leg, so as I could work out what the pain was? He contemplated this question for a few seconds and then rolled onto his back and said, "Okay, no-one else has been able to help me, so you may as well try!" I then requested if the student nurses could come into the room, so I proceeded to ask Mr Finch if he was happy to have them there? He nodded yes, they then entered, closing the door behind them.

"Mr Finch, can you point to where the pain is?" I asked. He pointed to his upper calf, so I then asked if I could have a look? He nodded, so I raised the head of the bed to make Mr Finch comfortable, then I raised the entire bed so I could visualize this area well after gaining his consent and informing him I was about to raise his bed. After gently exposing the calf by pulling his pyjama leg up, I could see quite clearly the problem. Mr Finch had an indwelling catheter, which was attached to a leg bag. The leg bag was secured to his upper calf with a velcro band. This white velcro band appeared deeply embedded into his flesh of the upper calf, so embedded in fact that it was forming a tourniquet around his lower leg. By loosening this velcro band, I immediately noticed a deep pink band of flesh left behind where the band had caused pressure. The relief Mr Finch felt from me releasing this tourniquet was immediate as he let out a huge sigh. He reached down to rub the choked area with his hand. He looked straight at me and smiled, as his pain was gone like that! Replacing that strained, agitated mood was a relaxed and genuinely grateful gentleman.

To my surprise, when I checked the medication chart, I found that Mr Finch had been given strong analgesic that morning. No-one had looked at where the pain was originating from, or where his leg bag was secured too tightly. I again checked the reddened area where the velcro had been and found the skin was quickly returning to its normal colour.

I then proceeded to ask Mr Finch the remainder of the pain assessment questions to complete the assessment thoroughly when assessing any pain or discomfort:

'Are you in any pain at present?'

'Can you point to the pain with one finger?'

Can you tell me exactly what the pain feels like?'

'Is it there all the time, or does it come and go? When did the pain start? Have you had it before?'

'Does it radiate anywhere?

'What helps relieve the pain?'

'What makes the pain worse?'

'On a scale of 0 being no pain, and 10 being the most pain you have ever had, can you tell me what number your pain is now?'

If the client has any pain, think of immediate measures that can help relieve this pain; for example, positioning, heat packs, gentle massage, quiet environment. Reassure patient. It's important to know what sort of pain they are experiencing. Is it a headache? Are they dehydrated? Stressed? Vital signs must be accurately done when a patient is in pain and examined closely for any changes/variations. Pain must be treated immediately. The area must be visualised and assessed thoroughly. If analgesic is given, reassessment of that pain must be followed up in a timely manner to ensure the analgesic is effective in treating their pain. Chest pain should be escalated to a MET (Medical Emergency Team) call to ensure immediate action is taken and as their nurse, stay with that patient until the chest pain is completely relieved. Different analgesics work for different types of pain. Is it nerve pain? Headache? Muscular? Wound pain? A developing pressure area? Angina? Something that can be relieved immediately? Mr Finch's pain could have been avoided by ensuring it was fastened securely, but not tightly and checking regularly on the leg to ensure it was not compromising skin integrity or circulation. Mr Finch was suffering! This pain was making him frustrated, sore and agitated. When someone is in this state, often pain is the source of this. People may not complain as they don't want to 'annoy' the busy nurses, so they put up with it, even when pain is a sign that something is not right. Pain cannot be questioned. It's important to emphasise to all patients that if they have any pain at all, to please notify a nurse straight away. Reassure all patients that it is no trouble at all and that you would rather be called straight away to ensure they are comfortable. Too often nurses underestimate the importance of thorough and regular pain assessments. Learning this essential skill as a student nurse is vital in your role to ensure all patients in your care are supported fully.

Mr Finch was always a gentleman who never spoke badly about anyone. His response was directly due to the pain he was suffering. He was agitated and fed up with it. Therefore, it is important to know your patients well and develop a close rapport with each and every one so that you can tell if a certain 'behaviour' is out of character for any person. Mr Finch had been constantly ringing his buzzer, not to be annoying or demanding but in the hope that someone would be able to help him. Fortunately for Mr Finch, his pain was finally fully relieved and quite quickly he returned to his usual, normal self. Pain is an indicator of something underlying. If a nurse fails to respond to this and thoroughly assess and act on this pain, the patient's condition could deteriorate rapidly. Analgesic could mask the pain if this pain is a sign of something more serious and it's not investigated thoroughly.

As a nurse we strive for optimal outcomes with all our patients. Never think that pain is trivial because pain can be like a scab but underneath the scab is a festering reason that pain exists. My students learnt a valuable lesson that day with Mr Finch that I am sure they will carry with them throughout their nursing profession. I still struggle to this day to see anyone suffering in pain. Never lose that deep compassion! If you do, you should really question whether you are in the right role. A nurse's most important quality I believe is one of deep compassion for our fellow human beings.

CHAPTER 5

Through A Childs Eyes

I have always had a soft spot for children. I seem to understand them, even before they develop comprehensive language. I can sense whether a child or baby is happy, angry, shy, confident, sad, suffering or content. Paediatric nursing was an area that I thoroughly enjoyed. I worked in a very dynamic, fast paced, ever-changing paediatric ward. These kids taught me so much about nursing and life.

Paediatric nursing involves caring for not just a sick/injured child but also caring for the parents. Play therapy is the most effective tool I developed in gaining that sense of trust. Calm, quiet environments are necessary and conducive to relax and heal a hospitalised child.

A child sponges off a parent's emotions. If the parent is sad, distressed, anxious, angry or scared, their child's emotions magnify these ten-fold.

This is where I learned that children, can deteriorate rapidly when unwell but also, they can do a remarkable turnaround and their health improve just as quickly.

Children I found were different to look after than adults in that their feelings and emotions were rawer and more innocent. They would cry and verbalise if unwell or in pain. I always knew that if a sick child was quiet and sleeping it was not always a good sign and my internal alarm bells would start ringing.

I worked on a ward that presented many challenges with our paediatric patients. You were often faced with very confronting situations when presenting for your shift. I take my hat off (and I love hats) to all those paediatric nurses out there who work tirelessly and often go home as I did, burying my head in the pillow from complete and utter exhaustion. Just to wake up and do it all again in the same selfless and compassionate professional manner as always.

I looked after many children who were very unwell, and they taught me more about living and dying than I ever realised at the time.

Many people as we get older, develop a genuine fear of our own mortality. Will death be painful? Scary? Lonely? But I looked after many much younger who knew they were dying and somehow appeared to accept their own mortality. I saw one young girl holding her mother in both arms as she was lying on her bed, her mother sobbing uncontrollably as she lay her head on her daughter's chest, listening to the sweet sound of her daughter's heartbeat. A sound that she knew in a short time would cease to exist. The young girl was stroking her mother's hair speaking calmly and softly, reassuring her grieving mother! "Mum, it's okay, don't be scared. I am not afraid." Indeed, she appeared to have a wisdom and maturity well beyond her given years that cannot be explained. She would draw beautiful pictures for her family with stick figures and houses and trees and rainbows and sunshine. Beyond the rainbow would be a figure she drew of herself, floating horizontally in the sky with wings and a big smile on her face. She spoke to me of her impending death and how her only concern was for her mother and family and how they would cope without her there. She epitomised the selfless act of acceptance of death and was at peace with death itself. Children are very smart and intuitive and in tune with their surroundings; they are honest and innocent and we should always be honest with them, listen carefully to them and allow them to express themselves no matter what form this may take – crying, drawing, playing and music. It is a privilege to nurse all children.

I reached hastily for the emergency buzzer as I felt the stiffening body of the little baby girl I had just been feeding. Just five minutes earlier I had changed her soaked nappy and prepared a bottle of breast milk her mother had left for her next feed. Her mum was exhausted and decided, after much reassurance from her evening nurse and paediatrician, that she would go home for the night for a much-needed sleep in her own bed whilst her baby girl stayed with us. Margot was an adorable baby with big brown eyes, her dark black eyelashes curled up, long and almost doll like. She smiled up at me as I approached her and reached into her cot to pick her up. I could see her cheeks, rosy and dimpled, glowing like rose petals. Her little hand like a starfish gripped onto my finger as I settled into the chair to bottle feed her. It was 2 am. I tested the milk on my inner wrist to make sure it was the correct temperature. I slipped the towelling bib over her head and she began sucking contentedly on her bottle. She was so relaxed and occasionally, as she studied my face intensely, she would smile and as the corners of her lips turned upwards, the seal her lips had created with the bottle would break and she found this quite amusing as the bubbles rose with gravity through the milk.

It was a lovely time of night, so quiet and it was important to have quality time when giving Margot her bottle. Margot had been admitted 3 nights earlier with "seizures" that had occurred at home. There were no apparent high temperatures associated with these seizures and Margot had been admitted for observation and investigation to try to ascertain the cause of these seizures.

Her little starfish hand reached up to touch my face gently as she gave me another precious smile. I took the bottle's teat gently out of her mouth, placing it in a container next to the bed when I felt her tiny frame stiffen whilst still on my lap. I reached the emergency buzzer on the wall easily and placed Margot gently in her cot as the cot side was already down. I quickly looked at my watch and started timing the length of the seizure. As people arrived to help, I watched Margot carefully for specific signs of this seizure. Her colour had changed from rosy pink to white. I feared she may aspirate, and I was glad I was so vigilant about checking the oxygen and suction equipment and that it was all in good working order at the commencement of my shift. Contents from her stomach could find its way into the lungs during a seizure as an unconscious person is unable to protect their airway and I was aware she had just consumed around 50ml of breast milk prior to this event. She was having a tonic-clonic (grand mal) seizure and this phase lasted about two minutes.

When able to, I lay Margot on her side to protect her from aspirating if she vomited but, thankfully, she was breathing normally again and required only a little oxygen therapy. Her colour returned quickly as she appeared to be in a deep sleep. Within a few more minutes she woke up and appeared sleepy and grizzly, but it wasn't long before she was back to her normal happy self, totally oblivious, thank goodness, to what had just occurred.

I was now observing her closely for further seizures and monitoring her neurological signs. My adrenaline was still pumping as we notified mum that her baby girl had just experienced a further seizure. Margot was still hungry, as she had not finished her bottle, so with the doctor's consent, I prepared another bottle for this hungry baby girl and she quickly took the bottle well and settled quickly into a deep sleep in her cot after being burped. I greeted mum as she arrived on the ward, naturally she appeared very concerned and was extremely worried for her little girl. I checked on Margot regularly and watched her closely for the rest of the night shift, ensuring her condition remained stable. I documented her seizure describing what had occurred on a timeline from the start to the completion of the seizure and what actions had been taken to ensure this child had a complete and thorough report of her seizure event and all care given was transcribed. Both the medical staff and I explained everything to mum so as she could be reassured that her child was going to be okay.

Margot underwent many tests over her next few days in hospital. She was diagnosed with Epilepsy after all the results were back. She underwent thorough investigations, an appropriate plan of treatment was undertaken and instigated by the neurology and health care team.

Margot was sent home after a few days and by this time her condition and medications were well understood by her parents. They felt safe and competent in managing her Epilepsy back at home.

I got to know Margot and her entire family well over the course of her stay and became very efficient at anticipating her needs. I ensured she settled well with her pink 'blankie' blanket. She hated being wrapped tightly. She would grizzle when hungry, rub her eyes and put her arms above her head when tired and coo herself to sleep. She liked to gently nuzzle into my neck when I was burping her and appeared to gain a great deal of comfort as I methodically patted her back. But when she woke from slumber, she would open her eyes so wide when she saw me and literally beam at me with a smile that melted my heart.

The day that she left the ward to go home, I felt complete happiness knowing that her quality of life was going to be really good from here on and she had every opportunity to have a normal and healthy life now, thanks to a team of people who were committed to give her the best care and advice available.

The reward you receive as a nurse is so much more valuable than monetary - it is to see an individual discharged from hospital happy and healthy and go back home to their loved ones. Nothing compares to this happy, fuzzy feeling I get every time I witness this. It makes it all worthwhile and it makes the tough times so worth it.

CHAPTER 6

Nurture Yourself

A s a modern-day nurse, it is our responsibility and duty to ensure that each and every situation we encounter, is dealt with the utmost respect, compassion and empathy we can muster. Nursing tends to make you realise to take nothing for granted.

It makes you really appreciate what you have. Your family and your friends are so cherished. Nursing also makes you value not so much material things, but the little things you experience and share, are worth so much more. The terms 'stop and smell the roses' and 'you don't live to work but work to live' are my mottos in life. Another favourite is 'charity begins at home'. 'How can you give to others, when you don't give first and fundamentally to your family or loved ones? Or 'how can you help others, who are 'drowning' if your own boat has holes in it and you are drowning yourself?' Nurses need to look after themselves to meet the demanding challenges faced in their day-to-day work. Being a shift worker can be exhausting. Working a late shift, followed by a morning shift, along with travelling to and from work allows you to develop strong organisational and work balance skills.

The necessity to be able to switch off when you leave work and to return again to apply yourself professionally, is an essential trait that is important to learn early in a nurse's career.

Throughout my nursing life, one thing has been observed over and over again. Nurses in all areas often fail to take their allocated lunch or tea breaks. Martyrdom is not a quality that is becoming in a nurse. If you believe it makes the individual nurse more professional or accountable or even more important, you are strongly deluded.

Nurses, physically and mentally, require their allocated breaks to rest and replenish. The role of a nurse requires you to be fully alert, to be able to deliver optimal care in diverse situations. I am not suggesting you take longer breaks than you are entitled to at all, but always ensure you hand over your patients thoroughly to a suitable nurse colleague. If a nurse agrees to care for your patients while a colleague takes their break, the nurse must care for those patients as well as their own. So, if a nurse willingly agrees to care for another nurse's patients, they should be coping well with her own workload so they can allocate time to also care for these extra patients. If their workload is already saturated, they should never agree to take on this extra work and responsibility, even if only for an apparently short time.

CHAPTER 7

Where There Is Life, There Is Hope

Being a child of nature and growing up in the country, I have great respect for all living creatures. Nature has a way of ensuring the survival of the fittest which, over the course of my time here on earth, I have found and had many experiences with, and seen many examples of this phenomenon.

As a small, inquisitive little girl, I would peruse tree branches for nests. It wouldn't take me long to find one with my keen eyes and of course, I would be itching to get a closer look, I would scramble up the tree, flinging my skinny legs up high to hook them onto a branch, pulling myself up with my arms to sit on a branch so as I could closely observe the treasure this intricate nest would behold. I would sit gazing into the delicate, smooth, inner saucer-shaped sanctuary of the nest, marvelling at how soft and warm it appeared and how perfectly built it was; a strand of human hair, a feather or two, straw, twigs, fur like material, all woven delicately to construct a master-built home.

Inside there would often be a clutch of eggs that were perfectly formed like china or porcelain, some delicately speckled with brown or black flecks through differently coloured backgrounds, predominantly white, beige or even blue, my favourite colour is blue.

I could spend what seemed like only a few minutes to me but was probably a lot longer studying these eggs and nests. I knew which birds lived in each nest, how many eggs each nest held and when it was a 'safe' time to observe a nest by watching closely for the 'parent' bird to vacate it in search of food or water.

One warm summer evening, as the sun was starting to sink slowly into the horizon, I was playing knuckles under a massive tree, close to the house, when I felt an object fall and hit my left shoulder. It landed with a gentle thud in a clump of grass next to my leg. I was a little startled at first, as I was unaware of what had fallen on me but on glancing over to the object on the grass, I quickly realised it was a young nestling bird. It was still immature with pink delicate skin, almost transparent, its dark internal organs could be seen through the skin that appeared as fine as tissue paper. Its head was huge and floppy, looking around as it lay splayed out next to me, flat on its back, its feet waving in the air. The baby bird appeared to be distressed and shocked as its beak was slightly open and it was breathing very heavily, almost panting.

I believe the fall and subsequent thud had literally knocked the air out of this little chick's lungs. On closer inspection, I noticed its left foot appeared deformed. I gently scooped the chick up into my cupped hands to further examine the claws. I compared the left claw with the right claw, which had normally developed claw and nails. The left claw appeared fused together and instead of 3 forward facing toes and one toe facing backwards; its 3 forward toes were fused as one thick band, with no apparent toe at all facing backwards. This little pink chick was chirping loudly as it was obviously distressed. I immediately knew it must be returned to its nest, as I mistakenly thought it must have fallen out. I ever so carefully scaled the tree after locating the nest high above my head, the nest was tucked neatly in a branch fork. To my dismay the mother bird was watching me closely with her beady eye, focused in a death stare. Her black glossy feathers spread fully over the nest; her wings splayed out like a deck of cards trying to inconspicuously conceal her precious hidden treasures. When I continued to approach her, she suddenly took flight and was gone. I jumped, clinging tightly to the chick in one hand and a branch in the other. I just avoided falling, head-first from the tree. Now with the mother bird gone, I could see three more chicks, their beaks gaping open, hungrily anticipating a feed.

I could hear the mother calling out angrily close by, she was not happy at all. I managed to reach over, swaying side to side I released my grasp on the little chick that had survived the fall earlier. It plopped down gently into the nest. Satisfied it was safe now with its siblings, I retreated backwards on the branch until I reached the trunk of the tree. I stepped down onto each branch, like it was the rungs of a ladder, jumping the last three feet to the ground. I was so very chuffed with myself that I had managed to rescue the chick and save its life (or so I thought). I ran into the kitchen to devour my dinner, sharing my conquest with all my family at the dinner table. Shortly after dinner, I excused myself and ran out into the yard again, to visit the nest I had found earlier. As I ran over to the tree, I saw something on the ground that caught my eye and my heart sank, I realised it was the chick. I fell onto my knees in despair and reached out to gently encompass its fragile little body in my warm hands. The little chick was cold and lifeless, I was devastated to find it had been attacked and was bleeding profusely. As tears streamed down my face, I stroked the little bird's featherless head until my mum came out. She had heard me sobbing and had come to find me. I just peered up at her through tear-filled, blurry eyes, words were not needed.

I buried this little chick in a beautiful lace handkerchief; no expense was spared. I struggled to understand why the mother bird had tossed her defenceless chick out of its warm, safe nest. What did it matter that it had a deformed claw? It was still beautiful and precious. Just because it would never have been able to perch on a branch, due to its deformed claw, it would work it out. How could its own mother have been so heartless and cruel as to kill its own baby with its beak? I was six years old and I knew then that my calling in life was to make a difference. My calling was to care for the sick, injured or vulnerable. This leads me to tell you next about one of the most rewarding areas in my nursing career that I was so privileged to be involved in.

CHAPTER 8

Touched By An Angel

I opened the door of the room after I heard a voice say, "Come in". I entered to find a lady and man inside. I introduced myself to the young couple and shook their hands respectively as they reached them out to me. Marion had swollen red eyes as she studied me through them. Christian looked pale and tired as he sat back down and sunk into the chair next to the bed. Marion continued to unpack her overnight bag she had brought in with her as I laid my paperwork down on the over bed table.

It was always gut wrenching to see a couple arrive, being admitted for an unviable pregnancy or termination of pregnancy for medical reasons. Marion had already changed into her paisley nightgown before I'd entered and as I deftly organised the admission paperwork, she slipped into the bed under the bedclothes watching me intently.

I showed them the room first, how to use the call bell, reading light and TV, as these controls were on the one unit. I then demonstrated how to dial out on the phone. I showed them the bed control, how to raise and lower the head of the bed as desired. I went on to explain that I would be their nurse for the next 6 hours or so and if during this time, they needed anything at all, I would be there to assist them in any way I could.

I then proceeded with the routine admission paperwork. I checked all the details including name, address, contact number, date of birth and emergency contacts. Firstly, I knew the importance of ensuring all these important details were correct. I confirmed every detail with Marion and Christian, then proceeded to make an armband with all of Marion's details securely attached and asked her to please check it, showing her the armband before I was satisfied it was accurate. She confirmed this with a nod, so I placed the armband immediately on her wrist. I enquired as to whether she had any allergies? She replied softly that she had no allergies. I weighed Marion, documenting this on the observation chart as well as the drug charts and admission sheet. Then Marion was accompanied to the toilet as she felt she needed to use her bowels.

I was aware that Marion had seen her doctor the day prior. She was booked into her doctor for a routine appointment when her pregnancy test came back positive. Marion was excited, as this baby was unplanned, but certainly not unwanted. The obstetrician had ordered an ultrasound to confirm dates and blood tests to see how the pregnancy was progressing. The news was not good, and her blood results indicated her foetus was non-viable and the ultrasound failed to detect the baby's heartbeat.

Marion had not exactly meant to get pregnant. Her and Christian had met only 9 months before they got married. It was love at first site. Christian was a university student, studying law in the same class as Marion and he sat right in front of Marion each session. Marion would drop her pen or books in the hope that this red-headed, handsome man in front would pick up her belongings and 'bingo', notice her! Her plan worked a treat. As soon as he clapped eyes on Marion it was game over. Before the week was over, they had fallen head over heels in love and since then, they were inseparable. Their life had been a whirlwind with university, a lovely wedding and they had more recently bought their very first house together. This baby news had come as quite a shock, but they had shared the excitement and dreams for their future with family and friends happily, unable to contain their joy. Sharing this news was only natural. They were elated to be pregnant.

Marion was chatting away nervously, but obviously felt a sense of comfort in my presence. Suddenly she expressed the urgent need to use her bowels. It caught her breath unexpectedly. I assisted Marion to the toilet, where I had placed a green plastic receptacle into the toilet before Marion had arrived. I immediately recognised this urge Marion had, as a possible sign that the foetus was about to be expelled from its temporary home.

As Marion sat on the toilet, she was unusually silent, but I could see she was intently focused on what she was doing. She was staring ahead like she was in a trance, focusing, concentrating, holding her breath and then, I heard Marion let out a deep guttural moan. I saw fine moist beads of sweat, glistening on her furrowed forehead. I quietly spoke to Marion, asking her if she would like me to stay. She nodded to me, making eye contact as if she was imploring me not to leave. I assured her that I was not going anywhere, her shoulders instantly relaxed as I heard a gentle 'plod' into the receptacle.

There was no need for words, it was clear by Marion's gaze directly into my eyes, that she knew what had just happened. I reached over and gently wiped a warm, damp cloth across her forehead. When she was ready to stand up, I assisted her with one hand to rise and pulled her pants up with my other hand, discreetly placing a clean sanitary pad securely in them. Reassuringly, I then placed one arm around her waist, while holding her trembling hand in mine and gently accompanied her out of the bathroom, back to her bed.

Christian was sitting on the chair next to Marion, reaching over to cover his wife with warm blankets as she appeared pale and in shock. She then said to Christian, "I think the baby's gone!".

I spoke to Marion and Christian, quietly telling them that I would update them soon on the baby. I did my best to reassure them in a calm tone, whilst focusing first and foremost on Marion. I was keen to take Marion's vital signs, to ensure she was not bleeding too heavily. I immediately performed these duties, satisfied that Marion was progressing as expected and all was well from a nursing perspective. I ensured I kept Marion fasting to ensure she could be sent to theatre if the need arose

When Marion was settled, I explained to Christian and Marion that I would return shortly. I then walked into the bathroom and retrieved the receptacle from the toilet.

I covered the container with a clean material cloth and excused myself as I carefully carried the receptacle into another room. I told them I would be back shortly. I asked them to please buzz me if they needed anything. They thanked me as I left their room.

I walked into the pan-room, but I couldn't bring myself to look into the container in a pan room, it just didn't seem right. I walked out of the pan room, into another small room. I closed the door behind me and approached a bench area. I popped on some gloves and drew back the cloth I had over the container. There appeared to be a large blood clot, about the size of my palm. I gently touched the clot and saw an opaque perfectly formed foetus, cushioned within the soft dissolving clot surrounding it. I gently touched the clot to reveal a complete baby foetus. I was mesmerised by the beauty I was beholding. The foetus was glistening and almost luminescent in colour. You could virtually see through its tiny fragile body. It was around 3 inches long – the head was three quarters of an inch long, the body also three quarters of an inch in length and the legs were around another inch long. I looked closely in awe of its perfection. Tiny ribcage, perfect head, ears, eyes, nose and its tiny, perfect hand was close to its mouth, the thumb at the mouth as if it had been deriving comfort not long before, from sucking its thumb. The eyes were dark and large – closed as if sleeping. The delicate arms were both bent at the elbows at a 45-degree angle. I was overcome with sadness to think this beautiful creation would never have the chance to breathe air into that perfect ribcage and would never have the opportunity to feel its mother's sweet breath on its face, or use those precious legs to crawl, or walk, or run. Nor would it ever hold someone close, in those exquisite arms. I gently lifted this perfect creation and ever so gently wiped the baby clean. I said a prayer for the soul of the child, ensuring it was warm by cutting down a small flannelette cloth I had located within the hospital.

I tenderly wrapped the baby's delicate body in the clean cloth as I would wrap a newborn, full term baby. Its little head was exposed, little hands were clearly visible.

I would not leave this baby cold or naked, nor would I leave this baby unloved. This baby was very much wanted and loved by both parents and the least I could do is respect this tiny baby.

I left the tiny foetus safe and snug as I washed my hands after removing my gloves before stepping back into Marion and Christian's room.

They looked up as I entered, and I knew they wanted to know what I had found. I gently moved closer to them and in a quiet, calm voice, I explained to them that I had retrieved their baby and with this expected news, their tears ran freely and they hugged each other tightly as they cried for the loss of their precious baby. Their future dreams, that had occupied their thoughts prior to this event, were now vanished. When they were more rested, I asked them if they would like to see and hold their little one. Marion looked at me and said she couldn't bear to see the baby, as it would be too difficult for her. I explained to her that I completely understood but if she changed her mind, to let me know, I was here to help her in any way I possibly could. Marion looked exhausted as I completed a physical assessment, attended to her vital signs, got a warm rug from our blanket warmer and tucked her in leaving her safe and comfortable, hoping she would finally succumb to a much needed and well-deserved nap.

As I left the room, Christian followed me and as I reached the nurse's station, I turned around and saw him. He looked at me and asked me if it would be okay for him to see his baby. I gave him a reassuring nod and replied, "Of course, Christian." I led him to a quiet lounge area, where there was a small coffee table and chairs and asked him to wait there, for my return.

On my return I had his tiny baby wrapped in the soft, custom made blanket, holding on, ever so securely and safely in both my hands. He was seated with his head down deep in thought as I approached him. He looked up as I handed him his precious and perfect child. As he took his little one, the child lay lifeless in his massive hand snugly wrapped up, he stroked the baby's head and teardrops ran down his cheeks like water flooding down a windowpane. The droplets splashed on the little baby's blanket and head and he deftly and gently wiped them off. He then clumsily but carefully unwrapped the blanket and gazed down at the most perfect and beautiful sight. He stroked the baby's little arm and hand and he gasped, "Just so perfect and so beautiful!".

He took a good 5 minutes or so, just having precious time with his child, that he would treasure always We just sat in silence as Christian absorbed every second of this precious time, to hold his baby one last time.

Christian bent his head down and kissed the tiny head before him. He then proceeded to wrap the little one up, snugly in its blanket and handed his baby back to me.

We both rose and he then tapped me on both shoulders and said, "Where are your wings? Where do you hide them as you are an angel - I can't thank you enough". I didn't know how to respond to these kind words, so I said, "Thank you." I gently carried both Marion and Christians' child back to the room I had found for it to rest in and I really felt so honoured and privileged to be able to help a couple through this difficult time.

I returned to work the next day to find a much more rested and relaxed Marion. This pleased me. Christian arrived to take Marion home and I gave them a teddy bear to cuddle whenever they felt they needed some comfort. This of course would never replace their precious child. This was my first of many experiences with couples such as Marion and Christian and I guess the one thing I am grateful for, is how both times and opinions have changed and developed over the decades. So much support and care are now offered and available, that many parents never received in the past. To choose to hold and cherish and mourn their precious child is something every grieving parent has a right to do, if this is their wish.

CHAPTER 9

Fighting For Our Rights

This brings me to the important subject of 'professionalism'. Nursing has fought hard to become a recognised modern-day profession. From the 1850's, the Florence Nightingale Era – to our current modern role as a nurse, many significant changes have occurred that define us as a 'professional'.

When I started my training in the early 1980's, we were at the doctor's beck and call. When they arrived on the ward, the banter between the other nurses would abruptly halt and we would all rise to our feet and offer the doctor a chair. We would hand him his patients' files and always accompany him on his round, setting everything down and fetching equipment that he requested. Referring his patients onto other professionals at his request (I say his as the medical profession was predominantly male back then). We would never dare to call them by their Christian name. It was always Dr, and we almost "bowed" to them when they arrived.

Today, I find it very difficult to call a doctor by their christian name, even when they say, "Call me David or Harry or Tom". It was so ingrained into me during my training not to do this, that I have to constantly remind myself that it is okay. There are many women doctors in the medical profession, they are now recognized based on their merit, no longer treated as incompetent just because they are female. Male nurses are also entering the nursing profession in greater numbers which has been a welcomed addition to the nursing world.

The 1980's brought about sweeping changes in our fundamental role as a nurse throughout Australia, instigated by the Royal Australian Nursing Federation (Victorian Branch) secretary, who refused to bow down to the government in power during this period, who appeared to be hell-bent on reducing nurses' classification and pay rates. We would not back down and neither would the nurse's union. It was the year of 1986, I remember this time so vividly as I was still I was still training when nurses went out on an indefinite strike, leaving a skeletal staff across all hospitals in Victoria. This strike was in support of abolishing non-nursing duties, hoping to improve nurse-patient ratios, along with remuneration consistent with our line of work.

We were not going to be treated like handmaids any longer!

I was on an evening shift and as I looked out of the patient's window on the third floor onto the street below. I could see in the distance to the left, a large crowd of nurses, dressed in red t-shirts with red flags gathering next to the busy road. These nurses were predominantly women. Many dominant politicians were not happy at all with the kerfuffle this caused, but these women were not going to bow down and fade into the background again. Tents were pitched outside the grounds and I was proud to be within these ranks. They were in for the long haul – this strike lasted for 50 days. Many motorists would toot their horns in support of the nurses strike and I distinctly remember whilst working within the hospital during these long weeks, hearing a tooting horn, which would spur me on to push myself further during this difficult and demanding period to ensure all our patients, continued to receive the best care I could give.

Thousands of nurses on strike during this period were struggling, hungry, and unable in some cases to feed their families, let alone pay their bills. The media sensationalised the strike with headlines crying out, "Nurses are neglecting patients", yet I can personally vouch for the fact that those skeletal staff left, worked tirelessly to ensure all patients received the valuable care they required. In fact, the patients were behind us 100% as well. The government eventually caved in on 19th December and the nurses won, by receiving many conditions that they had initially asked for, finally persistence had paid off.

I guess, having been a part of this history, has really made me appreciate how hard and long we have worked for professional recognition in nursing.

I occasionally have undergraduate nurses arriving for clinical placement with multiple facial piercings, thick heavy makeup, inappropriate clothing showing too much cleavage and unsuitable footwear. I believe that presentation and being prepared for a nursing student is essential from the outset. For them to take a certain pride in their appearance and their conduct, including bringing a good attitude to work is paramount to how they will succeed in the nursing profession.

No matter what is going on in my life, when I go to work and step into my uniform, I leave all my troubles behind. For the people we are caring for require our focused and undivided attention. Each and every one, deserves our best care. We need to be there to listen, to meet their health needs. We need to guide them and educate them. They place their trust, and their lives in our hands. With every decision we make, it can improve their health. Never, ever should we attempt to do anything that could potentially 'harm'. If in doubt, stop, think and don't attempt anything unless you know how to do it and why you're doing it and what will happen when you do this. Troubleshooting and risk management are important to know before you perform any clinical skill.

Are you following the facility Policy and Procedures? If not, why not? These important guidelines protect foremost the patient, but also us, particularly when things don't go as expected or hoped for.

Always be prepared for the unexpected. Prepare everything prior to delivering any clinical skill. Explain what you are doing to your patient and listen to their questions, fears and comments. If they do not want something done, it is important to educate them on why/how that task will help them. If they still refuse, we respect their wishes and do not perform the task, then we should notify their doctor.

Informed consent is essential with every single task we perform, every day. It is their body; it is their right to refuse too. When you are writing your nursing progress notes, it should be mentioned that you obtained informed verbal/written consent prior to performing a task. It was carried out according to the facilities policy and procedure, for example: "Administering blood and blood products Policy'. Document if it went smoothly, or if there were any untoward effects and what action was taken to deal with these. Record the outcome of this action. Review with any follow up tasks. It should be factual, timely, orderly, clear and concise, giving a thorough timeline of all tasks performed.

CHAPTER 10

Are My Shoulders Strong Enough To Bear This Burden Of Responsibility?

As I woke up in my bed, I realised it must be late afternoon, or even early morning? There was a milky light of day coming through my curtains, so I reached for my phone next to my bed. I strained to see the time through my puffy eyes which were struggling to see and focus clearly in the dim light. It was 6:10 pm!

I panicked for a minute, I thought momentarily that I might have slept in. I had been on night shift, but my racing heart settled when I realised that I was rostered off tonight. As I sank back into my soft pillow, the reality of the events the night before, came rushing back into my conscious mind and hit me with a wave of deep sadness.

Earlier in the evening the night before, I was doing my rounds, settling and checking on all my patients. The ward was full and busy as usual. There were only two of us working hard to attend to our patient's care and we had divided the ward in half to focus on our allocated patients.

I systematically attended to my patient's rooms. I prided myself in my organisational skills and attended to the usual nightly ritual of vital signs, pain assessments, administering night medications, panning and accompanying patients to the toilet and generally ensuring they were all warm, stable and pain-free. I was only interrupted a couple of times by a buzzer. I answered call bells promptly and then back to the task of ensuring all patients were stable, safe and comfortable.

Mr Smith was sprawled back on his pillow, reading the Herald Sun when I poked my head in to find out how his day was? His spectacles were propped up on the end of his nose as he diverted his gaze up from the newspaper he was reading to give me a smile.

"Good evening", he said in a cheery voice. I proceeded to wash my hands and take his vital signs as we chatted away about how his day had been.

He was one day post-operatively and had undergone abdominal surgery. His vital signs were all within acceptable limits. No fever (afebrile), normotensive (blood pressure was stable), I felt his pulse radially, it was regular, rate was 84 beats per minute and his respiratory status was 16 breaths per minute, resting and breathing up well. His oxygen saturation from his finger probe was 98% on room air. His colour was also good. He was warm, snuggled under his blanket. His peripheral circulation indicated he was well perfused as both his hands and his feet were pink and warm to touch.

I asked him if he had been up taking gentle walks. He said he had been sitting out of bed and he had wandered around the ward on many occasions during the day. I then reminded him to wriggle his toes, roll his ankles and bend his knees to help improve the blood flow when lying in bed or sitting. This was to help prevent the development of clots. I educated him on the importance of continuing gentle ambulation and doing these active exercises until he resumed full activity after he went home.

Mr Smith was to be discharged from hospital the next day, so I took the opportunity to educate him of important information related to his ongoing care once home. Prevention of DVT (deep venous thrombosis) was an important subject to discuss with all of my patients from pre-operatively, when they arrived in hospital until well after they went home, as there were increased risks of DVT developing due to surgery, hospitalisation or any illness or situation where they are not as mobile as usual.

Back in the 1980's, DVT prevention was still important but compared to today with increased knowledge and technology, advanced by leaps and bounds in this area, such as use of anti-embolic stockings, correctly sized and fitted for all abdominal and high-risk surgery. Use of sequential calf stimulators pre-surgery which remain on when patient was post-operative and resting in bed, prophylactic prescribing of anti-coagulants (blood thinners) by attending doctor if required. Checklists of determining risk of DVT are done regularly by nurses to ensure DVT prevention strategies are in place to help prevent DVTs from occurring. I then checked that Mr Smith's discharge medications had been sent to the pharmacy. It was all green lights for Mr Smith heading home the next morning.

I then asked Mr Smith if he had pain? He said his pain was minimal, so I conducted a full pain assessment whilst he was reclined back in his bed. He pointed to his fresh abdominal scar when I asked him to point to his pain. He described it as a little 'stingy' and 'itchy'. "Itchy" was an adjective often used to describe a healing wound, as indeed Mr Smith's post-surgical wound was. After conducting a full pain assessment, I was satisfied the pain being felt by Mr Smith was wound pain.

I asked Mr Smith if he would like some analgesic to help relieve his pain. He nodded his head; he looked settled, so I gave him appropriate analgesic, which had been written up for him post- operatively. I made sure his buzzer was close and he was warm. I wished him goodnight and asked him to buzz me if he needed anything at all.

The ward was so quiet. It was 11:00 pm and you could have heard a pin drop, but I wasn't complaining as there was lots of fluid balance charts to tally up for the day to keep me busy. It gave me time to do these before midnight. I quickly got them done in around 35 minutes, then picked up the torch to check on my patients in the "back area". This was the area behind the nurse's station. It was the area where there were single rooms, so this area was often used to place terminally ill or infectious people who could really benefit from the solace of a room on their own. The back area was full of different patients tonight, most of whom had been to theatre and would be going home in the next few days.

As I walked into Mr Smith's room, my hairs stood up on my arms. Immediately I could sense something was not right. Call it my gut instinct or just plain pure sixth sense, but I felt it strongly at that precise moment I walked into his room, I shone the torch from my feet to Mr Smith's bed. I had a sickening feeling in my stomach as my pace quickened and my torch began to scan the bed where Mr Smith lay.

Mr Smith was on his side, seemingly peaceful and sleeping, however when I looked at his face he was as white as a sheet, his eyes were open, and he was staring straight ahead. I touched his arm and called out his name, all the time knowing that Mr Smith was not asleep, but he had in fact passed away. He was not breathing, his chest was not rising and falling, he was not responding to me calling his name. My heart was pounding loudly as I looked for any obstruction in his mouth and then called for help. I rang the emergency buzzer as I continued to prepare Mr Smith for cardiopulmonary resuscitation. As they say, time stood still as the room filled with people who took over their various roles.

Communication was good between these people. It was clear and concise. Doctors were contacted promptly. Mr Smith was intubated by an attending anaesthetist but despite being given all care available ... Mr Smith failed to respond to all resuscitation attempts. Every minute felt like an hour to me. It was as if everyone was moving in slow motion during this resuscitation effort. I looked on and felt helpless. I assisted with cardiac compressions, obtaining ongoing absent signs of life, despite an extraordinary effort on behalf of all the health team. It was futile.

Mr Smith had left his lifeless body and could not be brought back. At 01:15 hrs his doctor who was covering for surgical that night called Mr Smith's time of death in a loud, firm voice. I peered out over the bed where Mr Smith was, and glanced through the open blinds at the streetlights, which were stretched out in the dark background of the Melbourne night, some occasionally blinking. My heart felt so heavy as I refocused my gaze back into the room where my precious patient, recently full of life, was now still and void of any signs of the wonderful man he was just a few hours ago. My eyes wept freely and unashamedly for my precious patient.

His family arrived and as I walked with them into his room, I heard a high-pitched wail pierce my eardrums as his loving wife collapsed on his bed, sobbing uncontrollably, her body wracked with grief.

It was as if I was in automatic mode the rest of the shift. I attended to Mr Smith and his family. He looked beautiful after his wash and shave. I splashed some of his favourite cologne on his cheeks. I spoke to him, as if he were still alive. The remainder of the shift went quickly and smoothly, but I was in total shock and at knock off time, I walked off the ward, saying to myself clearly, "I will never come back here or nurse again!"

I was a broken girl. As I drove home, I felt like a failure. What was my purpose as a nurse if I couldn't help my patient? My mind kept going back to earlier in the evening when I last saw Mr Smith. Did I miss something? Could I have done more? What happened? I went over every minute detail of my time with Mr Smith and there was nothing I could find that indicated that anything was wrong. I felt so personally responsible for what had happened to him and began to seriously lose faith in my ability to nurse. How could I possibly continue with this profession I thought I loved after this? Could I continue to nurse if there was the possibility of this ever happening again? Was I cut out for this profession?

I got home, stripped off my work clothes which fell into a messy pile on the bathroom floor and took a long hot shower. I was in a daze, exhausted both emotionally and physically and only mentally woke up when the water ran cold and I was shivering. I managed to dry myself off, crawling into bed with my hair dripping wet. I was drifting in and out of sleep, but my mind was just focused on dear Mr Smith and his grieving family. My pillow was damp, not only from my hair, but from the warm, salty tears I cried, until sleep enveloped me and took me into an empty world of dark nothingness.

I really don't know how I got out of bed later that day. Nor how I managed to walk back into work a few days later, as I had lost my mojo. It took a massive effort to put my uniform back on and even feel like a nurse, but I did.

I gained the courage from somewhere deep within to face another shift and take on the responsibility of another patient. I realised now the immense accountability that comes with calling myself a nurse and this tragic event gave me an almost insatiable appetite to know even more about everything I did, to ensure I always gave the best care I could. Not that I hadn't felt this was important before, but the term "accountability" had more meaning than ever before.

A few weeks later I overheard two doctors discussing Mr Smith's autopsy results and the findings were that he had died from a large myocardial infarction. I was shocked to hear this. I thought I may have seen some obvious signs of such a thing as a heart attack. But it had come out of the blue, with no apparent clinical signs at all. All I hoped was that he didn't suffer. That it was so quick he never felt pain, or knew he was dying. I guess I will never know these answers. But one thing I do know, is that I could have walked away quite easily from my chosen profession after Mr Smith had passed away due to fear and uncertainty and, to be honest, lack of professional support. I wasn't one to go home and speak of my work to family or friends, as it was just something I never wanted to do.

Nowadays it has been recognized that it is imperative to attend an incident debriefing immediately or as soon after the incident occurs as possible. It may not necessarily even be a death, but an incident at work that may disturb a nurse to the point that the nurse may develop a fear, or it may be that it is on their mind a lot. Maybe they cannot sleep, as this incident keeps playing over and over in their mind. This needs to be recognized by the individual and they should seek out professional help to assist them in dealing with this event, so they can learn to move forward in a positive manner professionally.

Post-traumatic stress can occur in nurses, along with other professions who work in similar stressful environments and if left untreated it can lead to dire and adverse outcomes which may lead to us 'burning out' in our professional role. I often speak to my student nurses about 'self-care'. It is vital for us to realise we need to be both mentally and physically strong and focused to help others who are sick and vulnerable. If we are struggling, we are in no condition to be caring for our patients who are relying on us to be consistent and focused on offering them the most optimal care we can provide to return them to good health.

Not all of our patients can be saved. For so long I wished I had a magic wand as a nurse, so I could cure all for my patients, like Mr Smith. But unfortunately, death too, sometimes is a sad but inevitable outcome.

If indeed I had walked away from the shift after Mr Smith died, I would have done a great injustice. I would not have made a huge difference every single day to someone in need of my care. Just to help relieve someone's pain, offer comfort to someone alone and dying, or to rejoice with a patient when they receive good news about their health … just to make them a hot cuppa and listen to them in the middle of the night … it is often the small things that mean the most … that touch a soul, that makes the difference and makes being a nurse so worthwhile.

CHAPTER 11

If At First You Don't Succeed, Try Something New

I always wanted to be a midwife. To deliver babies and work with them every single day seemed to me like it would be the ideal job! So, when I finished my training and spent some interesting time working in theatre, I applied for a midwifery training position at a 'sister' hospital to where I trained. I was nervous when I applied, but confident in the fact that I would get this position I so dearly wanted. Not getting it, never even crossed my mind. I was always the eternal optimist and I still am. I dressed in a skirt suit which was a soft pastel orange in colour, with a crisp collared, broderie anglaise, long-sleeved, cream coloured shirt, with matching sensible cream shoes and 'natural tan' stockings.

I had achieved an excellent result for my final exams in nursing. I was a natural, to be a midwife, or so I thought.

I arrived early for my interview and checked in with the Director of Nursing's receptionist who showed me to a waiting area outside her office, where there were 3 large timber chairs with soft cushioned upholstery. I sat in one feeling very regal and not out of place at all. I was dressed like a tailor's dummy. My hair was long but pulled back from the sides and clasped at the back and I didn't wear much make up as my tan was golden, I dearly wished to make a good impression. Finally, the door creaked open and a head peered around to call my name. My heart was beating out of my chest, I could barely hear, due to its' resounding "lub-dub" beating loudly in my eardrums. I stood up and felt very self-conscious as I smoothed my hand over the back of my skirt to check it was sitting properly.

I entered the room, finding two ladies sitting, facing me behind an oversized mahogany desk. They peered at me over their spectacles as I smiled to greet them. They gestured for me to sit. I thanked them and sat crossed legged on the large upholstered chair which seemed to envelope me as I sunk further and further down into it. It felt deliciously comfortable, much like it was made of soft putty. I answered their questions honestly and thoroughly. I was so self-assured, by the end of this interview, I just knew I had done well. They scribbled in their books while I sat in complete silence. The ladies farewelled and thanked me, informing me they would be in touch shortly with their decision.

I went about my everyday activities that week, reassured that I had excelled in the interview and would soon be studying midwifery, something I had long dreamt of.

On Thursday, exactly one week after I attended my interview, I received a formal looking white letter in the mail. I tore it open in excitement, not being able to control my enthusiasm. The letter read in bold black, stark print. "On this occasion you were not successful in your application for a place on the next midwifery course commencing in February 1987."

I just stared at the letter for a minute before I noticed a big wet tear had splashed on my letter, as I watched that tear run down the letter I started sobbing loudly, ran to my room, threw myself on the bed and cried my heart out.

I couldn't fathom why on earth I had not been accepted! Did they not like the colour of my skirt? Was I too confident in my answers? Did one of them not like me? I was completely devastated, as not being accepted was something I did not even consider. I thought it was a done deal, a definite outcome. Yet somehow, I know when I look back at this result, I realise now in hindsight, how this decision has changed the course of my entire life.

If I had been accepted, I would not have pursued a graduate year at a large public hospital closer to my home, where I learnt so much about many diverse areas in nursing. It broadened my scope to acquire a love for diverse nursing in cardiac, renal, neurology, spinal, high dependency gastro-intestinal, respiratory, medical and surgical care. I developed a love for adult nursing, but I was surprised when I worked on the paediatric ward how dearly I loved working in this busy ward, and this was to shape me into paediatric nursing for a good 12 years or so of my career. It was my love, it was my strength, it was my inspiration and I cherished every moment I spent there, giving all of myself.

I learned an invaluable lesson by not being accepted into the midwifery course. That is, life has a funny way of giving you not necessarily always what you want but gives you just what you need. Everything happens as it should, even when we don't understand how it could be good or right, it happens for the best.

A lot of good can come out of "bad" things. Maybe, just maybe, we don't always get what we want because there is something much better just waiting for us around the corner.

I trust in the universe now, as everything is as it should be.

If you reach out and help and give to others, your rewards are greater in giving than receiving. Happiness is the way we perceive what we have. If you value the simple things and treasure the important things you have such as family, health and friends, then you will be happy.

When I fail at something now, I don't feel a failure if I have done my best. It's just the universe telling me there is something better out there that will appreciate my talents and who I actually am. A place where I can shine.

CHAPTER 12

Life Is Precious And Fragile

I n the summer of 2014, I had a phone call one afternoon from my sisters, informing me my beloved brother John had died suddenly and unexpectedly. I was in shock. But I had to try to do what I could to help my broken, shell-shocked family and day by day, together, we got through the funeral and emptiness we all felt.

Mentally, I had appeared to survive this initial period of grieving for my precious brother, but physically my body was responding in its own way to this shock. I ceased menstruating, and about a month after John's funeral, my hemoglobin level had dropped, this was unusual as I had hemochromatosis, a condition whereby I normally had too much iron circulating, and I had venesections (blood taken from me and used as donor blood) to keep the extra iron from depositing in my major organs. Hemochromatosis is genetic. My mum was diagnosed 10 years earlier and I also had hemochromatosis. It was something I had learned to live with and control, to remain physically healthy. To have low hemoglobin was unusual, to say the least, so a general practitioner ordered iron tablets to rectify my anemia. Normally, I would have questioned this treatment and requested further investigations into why I had suddenly become anemic, but in my grieving state I didn't question or challenge my GP on this treatment.

Within a fortnight of commencing the iron tablets, I woke up one morning to left lower abdominal pain. I also felt exhausted, just like I had all my energy leeched out of me during the night. My temperature was sitting around 39 degrees Celsius My abdomen was gurgling and distended. I made an appointment to see my doctor who ordered a CT (computed tomography) scan and commenced me on Augmentin Duo medication. The CT scan confirmed I had Diverticulitis.

Wow! I had never imagined Diverticulitis could be so painful and that I could feel so very lousy with it! I remember patients being diagnosed with diverticulitis and I thought that it wasn't much, just pouches that had formed in the bowel, causing inflammation in these weakened pockets. I felt guilty that I had never acknowledged this illness and understood it more thoroughly before now.

I just blew it off as "nothing much" and boy, was I wrong!

Over the next 4 years, I had frequent flare-ups which became severe as the years went by, often ending up hospitalized as my bowel wall would inflame and leak causing micro-perforations into my peritoneum.

On my MRI scan, it was apparent my affected bowel was developing a thickness due to the toxicity poisoning my system causing scar tissue. In 2018, I found with each attack it was taking longer to recover, up to 3 months and even when I thought I was feeling well, as shown during a colonoscopy I had in April 2018, it was still inflamed long after an attack.

After much deliberation and lengthy discussions between my wonderful, well-respected surgeon and I, the plan was to ensure I was as well as possible, the aim was to try to get my inflamed diseased bowel to optimal health and that would be the ideal time to operate. This operation would aim to remove the offending diverticulum, and all the bowel it occupied from my rectum, to my sigmoid colon, to up north, past my splenic flexure (in large bowel). It was major surgery, but it was an opportunity for me to never have diverticulitis again, this was the desired goal. To be able to live my life. To travel to places where I would never be able to go with this awful disease. To commit myself to work, without the fear of me suffering diverticulitis and not being able to fulfill this commitment. I desperately wanted to be well again!

For years now I had been behind par with no energy as my gut had slowly been leaking through these pouches into my sterile peritoneum. I never felt good, always nauseated. My stomach was swollen the majority of the time and it was not uncommon for me to have pearly sweat beads surface on my smooth forehead. Nobody really understood just how debilitating this disease was for me. I wanted a chance to feel truly alive again. I was a good 54-year-old and although I was scared at having such major surgery, I really had no choice if I wanted some quality of life for the future. Finally, a date was set; June 4th was" D" Day.

I prayed I would stay well to be able to undergo this surgery. An anterior resection was booked in and it was only 3 weeks away but seemed forever to wait.

My mum, who was the grand age of 94, had a perforated diverticulum in her 50's, and thanks to wonderful doctors, surgeons and hospital she survived this dire, life-threatening emergency. Mum's perforation was sudden and deadly, peritonitis developed quickly, and she was rushed to theatre, her abdomen was cut straight down the middle and her large bowel where the diverticulitis was resected and removed. Faecal content had spilled into the peritoneum around all of mum's vital organs and this had to be thoroughly washed and cleaned out after rejoining her bowels before closing mum's abdominal wound. Mum was in ICU for a good week on antibiotics and it was touch and go for quite a while during this critical time. She survived this terrible illness.

I knew that if I did not have a bowel resection to remove my diseased part of my large bowel, I too would perforate. Deep down I knew that I must undergo an elective bowel resection at the most optimal time to eliminate the risk of perforating and have the most optimal outcome.

I was very much like my mum it seemed genetically, but my nature and personality were perhaps more like my father who had died back in 1998. He was relatively carefree and a happy go lucky nature, mum was more of a warrior. She was concerned for me having this surgery as she knew and remembered well the pain and risks this surgery had. Mum wasn't looking forward to her youngest born having this operation, but I felt I was facing a bullet to my head either way.

I could choose to ignore these signs and allow it to hit me unexpectedly and totally unprepared in the hope that the damage was repairable, or I could prepare myself both physically and mentally, then plan this assault, so the damage could be more predictable and less deadly. This was my chosen course of action and to be honest the wait until 4th June was long and frustrating. I prayed I stayed well with no flare-ups so the surgery could proceed as planned.

CHAPTER 13

"D" Day

I t was a dreary cold Monday morning. I was dressed in a crisp white hospital gown tied in two places, mid back and bottom, with nothing much on underneath but my pale pink, bare birthday suit. My sister sat in the high-backed chair in front of the window, which rose 7 floors above the inner city. Views were seen in the distance to the bay, which was grey in colour today, and people in cars, trams and on foot scurried along like ants from up here.

My daughter sat next to her, peering at me with a concerned look as I lay in the white cotton sheeted bed with my legs stretched out but casually crossed, displaying white anti-embolic stockings which clung to my calves and lower legs up to the knees.

I was ready and waiting to be called down to theatre, just when my sister's phone rang and she pounced on it answering it with a concerned, "Hello mum. No, she's still here." My mum was waiting to hear from my sister when I went in and anxiously asked her carer's in her aged care home to call Jane for an update as she thought I'd have gone in by now.

I bid my mum goodbye and as I was about to end the call, she blessed me and told me she loved me for the third time that day.

Just minutes after I hung up from mum, two people entered my room to take me down to theatre on my bed. It was now time to say goodbye to my sister Jane and my daughter Amanda. Goodbyes are always so fast. With a hug and a kiss, I was swept away on my hospital bed. Lying flat on my back, watching the roof go by, this way, that passageway, then finally in the lift. It was like an 'out of body' experience. I know I was there as large as life but those around me were chatting away above me. It was at this stage I felt insignificant and almost invisible.

I also felt this complete sense of helplessness. I was scared out of my wits, yet if I had of wanted to run, my legs couldn't have helped me flee, but my mind had been made up. I had to go through with this surgery now no matter what, if I had any chance of wanting a better future for myself. I just watched the people above, chatting away over the top of me, oblivious to the fact I was still there beneath them ….

Then we arrived on the theatre floor and I heard someone say I was the 'anterior resection' on the afternoon list as my bed was pushed into a corner. After a few minutes a lady came up to me and introduced herself as 'Peggy' the anesthetic nurse. Peggy went on to inform me that she would be assisting the anesthetist and would be by my side for the entire procedure. I felt my arm reach out in a gesture of pure fear to hold her hand and said, "Thank you Peggy."

I was wheeled to a little room outside theatre, where I had the anesthetist approach me. He popped a 'drip' (intravenous cannula) into my left wrist and administered some medication through this, a wave of giddiness swept suddenly over me, I was comfortably drifting in and out of sweet slumber, with not a care in the world. I remember when I woke, still waiting outside the theatre doors, partially peering through glass, which indicated to me enough to know that the 'quick' colonoscopy prior to my procedure had been lengthened due to unforeseen circumstances. Needless to say, by the time my anesthetist returned to me I was literally 'bursting' to go to the toilet.

I looked at him and he asked me if I could hold on until I was under anaesthetic as a catheter was to be inserted for the surgery and post-operative period. I was happy with this. I really remember little more. I cannot even remember being wheeled into the theatre. I just remember a dark nothingness for the next 5 hours ... it seemed like seconds before I heard voices in the darkness as I was coming out of this world of peace. I remember voices and was acutely aware of my mouth feeling as parched and dry as nothing I had felt before. This dryness extended well down my throat and into the entrance to my lungs where it felt almost raw and swollen. I swallowed painfully as I opened my eyelids. The first words I uttered were to ask for a drink of water as I muttered 'my mouth feels like the bottom of a birdcage'.

I drank the cold delicious glass of water down in a few gulps and it hardly quenched the deep thirst I was suffering. I have no recollection of waking up at all in recovery. I realized that my first moment of awareness was outside my room as I was being wheeled back into my room on the ward. I felt a kiss on my cheek as I opened my eyes, to see the most beautiful sight ever, my precious daughter Amanda before me looking concerned and placing something soft under my chin to comfort me. It was a little yellow teddy she had purchased to cuddle and keep me company whilst I was recuperating in hospital (so I found out afterwards) as I was too out of it to realize what it was at the time. My gorgeous sister Jane was there also when I awoke. She told me it was all over and that it had gone well, and he had 'got it all' (referring to the diseased area of my bowel).

My surgeon had popped in to see Jane and Amanda, when I was still asleep in the recovery room to let them know that the operation was over, and successful! Apparently, he had spoken to me also in the recovery room, informing me how the operation had gone, but to this day I still remember nothing of his chat, or even seeing him in recovery. It is amazing the power of medication and the effects it has on both the mind and body of an individual.

I have such a great respect for medication that it is given in correct doses and used for the sole purpose of alleviating pain or suffering in the correct manner that it was meant and made for. It is a wonderful tool when used with correct precision and can make such situations more tolerable and pleasant. I consider the role of the anaesthetist perhaps the most important role in surgery, other than the surgeon's job of course. The anesthetist has your life in his hands and putting someone to sleep, then most importantly, waking them up again is a great responsibility!

I often think, as I am being put under anaesthetic, if the worst happened and you were never to wake up again, you wouldn't have a worry in the world. It is a very peaceful and beautiful sleep that equates to no other sleep I have felt before. It is important to place your trust into both your surgeon and anesthetist's hands. It is important to relax knowing you are in good hands. For me, as a registered nurse, relinquishing all responsibility and healthcare duties was essential now for a full recovery.

Speaking of pain. Personally, I have always felt I had a high pain threshold. When I was admitted to hospital with diverticulitis and micro-perforations, I was often unable to stand up straight due to being bent over in pain. However, I was still reluctant to take anything (analgesia) for pain. The reason being, that I was not trying to be a hero, I felt strongly though, that I did not want to mask the pain I had with analgesia as this pain was an indication to me as to whether my condition was worsening (when pain increased) or whether my condition was improving (when my pain naturally subsided). My fear was that I would perforate and not recognize this until it was too late, if it was masked with pain relief. It made sense to me that once I had commenced on antibiotics, my pain ideally should gradually improve without analgesia. This was a good indication that my diverticulitis was settling down again.

My fear of becoming constipated and exacerbating the inflammation in my bowel if I took many opioid analgesics was real. Hence, I steered clear of all opioid/codeine-based analgesia and anti-inflammatory medications as I did not want to upset my gut any more than it already was. Post-operatively, I really had a mindset that I would be able to 'tough out' the pain. I was dreaming. As I attempted to move up the bed myself, I thought my abdomen was about to pop open there and then as the depth of pain I felt was like a hot knife piercing deep inside me.

I knew the importance of deep breathing and coughing to prevent atelectasis (collapse of part of the lung) from occurring so I propped a pillow up against my tummy and managed to cough very tentatively. I remember my anesthetist informing me I would require regular opioids, but I really didn't think that this would be the case for me. Was I wrong!

By the time my next pain relief was due, I was ready and willing to take the analgesia, as it was probably the only way I managed to get moving so early after theatre.

Perhaps the worst part of the first night was that I suffered from the most severe indigestion and reflux I had ever experienced in my life! I informed my lovely night nurse and she phoned the anesthetist who ordered something to relieve my reflux. I also asked for the head of my bed to be elevated too. I am sure it was elevated close to a 90-degree angle, so I sat bolt upright all through the night.

With hourly catheter measurements being taken and an intravenous pump chugging away in the quietness of the night, I managed to drift off nicely in between the myriad of vital signs that were taken routinely. Overall, I can look back and conclude that the first night was indeed, despite the pain, indigestion and disturbance, a lot more comfortable than I had dared to imagine it would be prior to my operation. I had been gifted back my quality of life and I will be forever grateful for my new lease on life.

CHAPTER 14

Recovery – On The Other Side

Yes, despite the building abdominal post-operative pain, I was so very happy. This pain was different to that of the pain I had felt almost constantly prior to my surgery. It was a pain I knew would improve with each day that passed. It was not accompanied by the exhaustion that came with my diverticulitis. I was free of that diseased portion of my bowel continuously poisoning my entire body. I felt instantly revived, energetic and I finally had hope again for a bright future where I could be me again. No longer lethargic and dragging myself along to do the most mundane tasks. I developed a new spring in my step and a twinkle in my eye that I hadn't experienced in years.

All my energies went into walking and learning to manage my new 'plumbing' down below. I swore then I would not become obsessed with my bowel activities, as I had witnessed in so many of my own patients. It was like I was a baby again, learning how to toilet myself as early on it was unpredictable, embarrassing, and windy! I remained positive it would resume a somewhat 'normal' routine with time and patience. With proper training, including diet and being close to a toilet in the early weeks, I, like a proud toddler, became adequately toilet trained again. After 8 weeks, all of my laparoscopic wounds had completely healed. I now believed I could finally look at getting back to the work I loved. I could finally travel without the fear of ending up in a strange hospital. It was good to be me!

I cannot begin to sing the praises highly enough of my wonderful surgeon, who guided me through this difficult but worthwhile journey for a better, brighter future for myself. He was not 'knife' happy and after seeing the loss of quality my life had become due to this debilitating disease, he discussed at each step, the best option, with each episode of diverticulitis. When I finally opted for surgery I was prepared as all avenues had been explored, including the risks involved. I could, god willing anticipate a positive outcome from this major surgery. I realized how lucky I was. I was surrounded on this colorectal ward by many others undergoing similar surgeries. Many had colon cancer and had not much time in which to prepare for the massive insult on their bodies when their bowel was removed and often joined again (anastomosed) with titanium.

Surgery has come a long way since I began nursing. Everyday more and more research is undertaken, more medical breakthroughs and ideas are discovered. Today, laparoscopic surgery has significantly improved outcomes, reducing complications, including infection, prolonged wound healing, adhesions and subsequently decreasing hospital stays dramatically.

I appreciated the nurses and doctors who took the time to explain things to me that I had never experienced personally before.

The day after my surgery I met a female surgeon who told me she had been assisting my doctor with my surgery. She gave me a first-hand account of exactly what had been done and mentioned that if I passed blood clots, not to be alarmed as this would be expected. My eldest son dropped in on his way home from work to visit me that evening. Midway through chatting, I felt something sticky run down my leg as I excused myself and ran to the toilet. As I sat there, I passed something sort of warm. When I looked into the toilet, I was shocked to see rather large old blood clots had been expelled from my bowel and I was quite fearful that I might begin to bleed. I presumed they came from the area where the titanium anastomosis had been created. I called out to my son through the partially opened toilet door, embarrassed with the strong, overwhelming smell wafting thick in the air. I told him it was best if he went home as I was scared that I would perhaps bleed more and didn't want him to panic and worry about me. I was so grateful to the resident doctor that she had prepared me for this. I was reassured that this was okay by the nurse, although she did pop a pan in the toilet in case I bled. A sensible thing to do I know, but it did make me feel a little uneasy. I thankfully did not bleed any further. I felt content that I was in good hands and was grateful for all the professional care, advice and information I received when I was on the other side.

CHAPTER 15

You Cannot Save Drowning People If Your Own Boat Is Leaking

A s I walked past his door each day, he greeted me with a big smile. There were many doors I walked past countless times as I was recuperating post-operatively in hospital but as I paced the hospital corridors and passageways, it was this gentleman who must have been in his late 80's that I constantly ran into. His name was Edward and I had seen him come back from theatre, with nurses and doctors constantly tending to him, watching him slowly progress each day to being able to sit up in bed, then sitting in his chair very tentatively. I saw this progress as I wandered on my daily walks, like looking into the pages of a picture book as I looked through the frame of his door each day, until eventually he escaped the confines of his room and the pages of his storybook. I was struggling to survive each day just like Edward, and although we would chat daily and have lengthy conversations about ourselves, I recognized the importance of my role as a patient, not a nurse to this lovely gentleman. He had been diagnosed with bowel cancer and was in shock, was scared and very frustrated and almost angry at times. I listened patiently to Edward and knew that I was not in the position to do much more. I too was a patient. I felt for Edward as he was desperately trying to come to terms with his illness. Listening was the best therapy I could offer. I was comforted to know that Edward was seeking and receiving not only the physical but emotional help he so desperately needed from the nurses and doctors on the ward.

I know that I was a fellow patient and also fighting to get well, I was no-where near strong enough, nor did I have the emotional energy required to support and help Edward. I was glad I was able to recognize this, as it was a necessary skill I had picked up early on in my nursing career. It has also helped to protect myself from getting burnt out in a profession where you are constantly giving. It is a profession where you learn to be grateful for the slightest improvement in your patient's condition, where a smile from a patient is all the thanks you need at the end of a long, hard shift. I have always learned not to get personally involved, no matter how deeply a situation can affect you. An invisible membrane must always be present so you can always manage to pick yourself up, seek the help you need, have a break and return as focused and strong as always. Otherwise bit-by-bit you will be eroded away. Then, you will not be able to give professionally your entire self to every new patient you look after. Your health and wellbeing are paramount if you are going to be the best nurse you can be. Nursing can be a lifelong and fulfilling career if you conduct yourself professionally every single day. Our vulnerable patients require this of us, so as they can receive the most optimal nursing care we can deliver in every situation.

If you cannot deal with pressures and move on and learn to be as, or more productive than before these challenges occurred, maybe nursing is not for you. I am not saying you shouldn't be sensitive, or you need to be hard. This is not the case at all, but you do learn to be sensitive, warm and compassionate but also learn to deal with lots of challenges, whilst always maintaining a high professional demeanor. To develop these qualities takes time, patience and experience and above all 'self-love'.

When you are starting out as a nurse you may become frustrated as you wish to do everything and be competent at all tasks. But with practice and focus and exposure to various experiences you will grow into your nursing role beautifully.

Good things take time to develop. Nursing is a career in which it will be forever changing and growing. There is always something new to learn with every situation. Don't ignore the small things, as 'A small leak will sink a great ship.'

Before you can grow professionally you need to be in tune with all the small things. Perform assessments thoroughly, document accurately, report promptly and follow each task through from start to finish, as those staff coming on after you will have plenty to do without having to complete half finished work. Of course, you only have one pair of hands so you will need to ensure you handover work you were just unable to complete. If a patient makes a request, do not say, "I will be back in a minute" and not go back to fulfil that request. Be a person of your word. Be transparent if you forget something, fess up and ensure you follow it through then. Apologize when this happens and if the client needs to wait, let them know they haven't been forgotten by offering them an explanation. This is respectful and thoughtful practice. Decent, honest communication is essential for a healthy nurse-patient relationship that is built on both trust and understanding. It helps make patients... more patient.

CHAPTER 16

Unexpected Occurrences

My day was going very smoothly. I had arrived early as usual, around 6:30am, checked staffing levels were adequate, allocated nurses to patients, checked on all night staff who were busy toileting, medicating and settling their patients after a busy night. It was busy with a full ward of both medical and surgical patients, but after checking on them by personally going to see them, I was satisfied they were all stable and comfortable.

Morning nurses came trickling into the ward from 6:40 am onwards. Doctors (physicians) and surgeons began arriving at around 6:55 am, so the night Associate Nurse Manager accompanied them respectively to their patients, giving the doctor a thorough summary of their current condition as they walked to their bedsides. I received handover at 7:00 am with the morning staff and quickly went to relieve the night nurse so as she could head home to her young family. I continued the doctors' round for the next few hours as I took orders, referred patients for specific tests and assisted doctors with whatever they required in caring for their patients.

A sweet looking lady was sitting near the nurse's station when morning tea was served. She sat comfortably with her overhead table in front of her. She had been showered and dressed, her hair washed, which was still damp but brushed back to one side, she had a part as straight as a soldier's back on the left side of her scalp. She peered out at the doctor I was accompanying, nodded her head and glanced at me, as I said, "Good morning Mrs. Clark!". I had never met this lady before as she had arrived on the ward late the night before but I had heard she had not slept well overnight and was quite loud and disruptive towards the other patients, so she had been placed on her bed in the passageway closer to the nurses' station to ensure she was safe and a closer eye could be kept on her.

The doctor's rounds had finally been completed and I was updating notes when I looked up from my paperwork as I was beckoned over to Mrs Clark by her finger. She had a smile that beamed all over her face and her eyes danced and glistened brightly as she said, "Excuse me dear, I have something to tell you", in a soft-toned gentle voice. I walked around the desk straight over to this lady who beckoned me to come even closer. As I leaned in to hear what she had to say, I just heard a clang and out of the corner of my left eye, I saw her hand move quickly and saw nothing else. I closed my eyes and just remember the pain of boiling hot, steaming water hitting my face. I remember gasping out loudly, but I must have cried out in shock as I recoiled from the pain. I felt my skin on my face, neck and chest on fire and I must have been too scared to open my eyes for what seemed like ages, but I am sure was only a few seconds. When I opened them and looked down on my chest to see my skin a fiery red, angry blushed colour, with white welts appearing as blisters forming almost before my eyes. My face felt almost swollen as it too felt like it was on fire. I stood motionless, unable to move or speak as the shock set in. Mrs Clarke had flung her boiling hot water from the jug for her tea at my face without any inclination of a warning and I was instantly in shock. By this time, staff were fussing around me, asking if I was okay. After a few minutes I pulled myself together and reassured them I was okay. I excused myself and went into the theatre where the showers were. I closed the door tightly behind me. I stripped off my clothes that were dripping wet as they were clinging to my scorched reddened skin.

I ran the water tepid, just cold enough for me to bear but not get a chill and stood under the shower with the water cascading coolly over my face, down my neck and onto my chest. I remember crying softly so as I could not be heard by others. It was like I hadn't cried for years following this, the quiet room suddenly filled with uncontrolled sobbing. I stood under that water for a good 15 minutes, hoping my eyes would not appear puffy and red from crying. When I stepped out of the shower, I dried myself with a towel I had grabbed on the way in and looked in the long mirror to check out the damage that had been done. It appeared like sunburn, uneven on the chest where the boiled water had trickled down through my clothes. I then put on a theatre top and pants that were cotton and somewhat soothing, they, loose and comfortable on my insulted skin. I dried off my hair and brushed it, as it was still damp on the blue cotton top.

I took some deep breaths, trying to gather my thoughts and make some sort of sense out of what had just happened. But there was no logic or rhyme or sense to be made. I stepped out back onto the ward, trying to act composed and get back into my work. Mrs Clarke had been moved back into her room. I was not angry with her. I was just shocked that I hadn't seen any "warning" signs to indicate that she was about to maim me with scolding water. It seemed she had calculated her actions carefully prior to this occurring – but I was totally oblivious and didn't hesitate to lean in to hear what she was saying.

Despite my wish to continue the shift, I was emotionally and mentally scarred and thankfully I recognized that I was not functioning in the capacity I needed to get through the shift. My physical wounds were one thing, but the emotional wounds were what really affected me. But that day, I learned a very good lesson. To always be ready for the unexpected and you must take good care of yourself before you can take care of others.

Any abuse in the workplace is not okay and the government has now taken a tough stance through the media and television ads that finally acknowledges the abuse healthcare workers face frequently in the workplace. No workplace is immune, and the abuse can be perpetrated not just by the public, or the patients or residents, but even by the staff themselves whose legal responsibility it is to protect their clients. There have been many cases highlighted of staff-resident abuse within our own aged care homes and these despicable acts have been caught on cameras often hidden in these residents' rooms. These acts of abuse toward their victims are criminal and these perpetrators when caught need to face up to the consequences of their words or actions.

I personally have been cussed, burnt, punched, kicked, slapped and spat on. I have had objects such as metal bed pans thrown at me full of urine and faecal matter. Despite this abuse, I have thankfully been able to return to work shortly after these incidents. They have not affected my ability to continue to provide the best care to all clients, regardless of their nature, physical or mental illness or capabilities.

Today people speak of "resilience". But when you are exposed to these abusive scenarios' day in, day out, how do you stop your resilience from being eroded away – until you simply say, "I cannot do this anymore!"

How do you prevent post-traumatic stress disorder from occurring? There are whole books on this subject and I am not about to make out I am an expert in this field as I am not, but I can say that I have found it helpful when I am exposed to traumatic events to recognize immediately the strong impact this event has had on me and seek immediate ways to deal with this personal stress. Debriefing of incidents should be organized in a timely manner and conducted by a professional who is trained to appropriately conduct these sessions. Follow up should be offered in the form of individual counselling and individuals should not hesitate to seek this out if they are not 'moving on' from an adverse event. Recognition and action are required by the individual to support their 'self-care', so they are able to remain physically, mentally and emotionally healthy. If we do not take this responsibility on and deal with it properly, it will affect our ability to function both professionally and also personally. Our personal wellbeing and balance are so important and cannot be overlooked or underestimated in our professional role. Simple things such as having meal breaks, switching off thoughts after work etc. will help you with 'self-care'.

Speak out and speak up to appropriate people in your professional environment if you are encountering a difficult situation with something or someone. Source the most appropriate people in your environment (usually a manager or supervisor) to discuss your concerns in a professional, private manner. Do not be scared or embarrassed or worried of what they might think of you as it is often things that you are most reluctant to discuss that concern you the most! Others may quite likely be having the same issues as you.

I believe to be resilient; you need to be honest and transparent. Speak out if it is important to you and acknowledge and face up to the things you feel. Always troubleshoot work issues with work colleagues to seek out better ways of dealing with these issues collaboratively.

I see resilience like a bouncing ball. When stressful situations occur, the ball is falling and hits the ground. Its ability to bounce back up depends on how we deal with this situation. The support we receive, our own health and wellbeing, how we perceive the situation, our attitude, whether we use it to learn from. If we do not deal with all these factors the ball may not bounce as high back to 'normality' leaving our coping mechanisms not as strong as before. After many repeated bounces, our ability to cope with each situation can decrease until … the ball fails to bounce back up at all. This affects us not only professionally but also personally and can destroy both the careers and lives of many wonderful people.

On this note, take care of each other. If you find a work colleague is a little 'off' offer your assistance and support this individual as we all have days where we do feel a little 'off' and it is nice to know our colleagues are there to support us and help during these times. We are all 'humans', 'unique' and 'diverse' individuals. No one is perfect. None of us know everything, we are all learning in nursing to do things an even better way. Sharing knowledge (preferably learnt through reputable research) is a great way to help optimize patient care. Collaborative work and interacting in a professionally caring manner with our colleagues, is the best way to improve our working environments and make it a positive, efficient and productive workplace. Personal work satisfaction is essential to grow and build professional confidence on. We all need to be recognized and valued for our hard work or our job can become very disheartening and you will quickly become 'burnt out' in your nursing profession. Stressful environments where strategies are not put in place to help staff deal with these stressors and where the support is not offered, find these places have a high turnover of staff and are also often less productive as staff morale is low.

It's not the winning that teaches you how to be resilient. It's the setbacks; it's the losses.

A lot of nurses I know today who have nursed for years are some of the most resilient people I know. They are not hard people at all, but they are firm believers that the harder the knocks, the stronger you can grow.

CHAPTER **17**

Rest In Peace My Friend

This story is about an inspiring nurse I was fortunate enough to not only work with - but to call my friend. Judy was a lady whom I met through work. She was from abroad and was in Australia to start a wonderful new life.

I often say it is important to develop therapeutic professional relationships and Judy was one I learned to really appreciate. She was always supportive. When the workload was great, she was the one you could always rely upon to get the job done properly.

She never complained but got into it, ensuring the job was carried out to the best of her ability. She would often ask if there was anything she could help with. I valued her teamwork and work integrity immensely. I appreciated her willingness and effort to take the time to make sure her patients were well looked after and she often spoke of the enjoyment she received when she developed trusting, positive interactions with those clients she cared for. She never bragged about her accomplishments, nor did she seek any accolades for her everyday work.

One thing I distinctly remember about dear Judy was her enjoyment and presence at work. She enjoyed all interactions, not only with her clients but also with her work colleagues and was able to step up when work demand increased.

She loved a chat and always had a smile when she was working. Judy went on to work at another facility and one day out of the blue, shortly after my brother had passed away she called me and informed me that she had found a workplace where she was really loving the work environment and was keen to get me back to work and on board after my brother's death. She mentioned how she had missed working with me and that she had spoken to the managers and they were interested in meeting me. Judy made me feel valued and appreciated, so before long I rang the facility and attended the interview. I was fortunate to be successful in securing a job in perhaps one of the happiest hospitals I had ever worked in! Yet again Judy and I were working alongside each other and it was always comforting to see her smiling face each day.

Judy often spoke of her beautiful home and how proud she was of it. She was always telling me about her garden and what her latest home project was. Home was her castle as far as I could tell!

Judy never complained about her partner at all, in fact she often spoke of how good he was to her. He bought her flowers and even organized 'surprise holidays' to enjoy together. I knew they had a few squabbles every now and again and time apart, but overall, she appeared bright and happy in her marriage, so I really didn't think any more of it.

Then one evening as I was watching the 6:00 pm news, I saw a photo of Judy come up on the big television screen and I couldn't believe what I was hearing. Something about Judy being found deceased and her partner had been taken in for questioning?! I was just staring at the television absolutely shocked to the core. It was like I was dreaming. This couldn't possibly be true! NOT JUDY! My phone then started ringing and it was work colleagues asking if I had seen the news about Judy. I just remember being in a daze, wandering around my house in disbelief, trying unsuccessfully to process what I had just found out. It surely couldn't be true; someone who was so vibrant, happy and full of life could not be just snatched away and gone like this!

That night, when sleep finally came to me, I dreamt I was looking down at her and her partner. They were arguing loudly, and it was as if there was a "fog" between them and I. However, I could clearly hear Judy yelling, "Stop! Stop! Stop!" and then – silence. I woke with a jolt, unable to go to sleep again that night as I was quite disturbed by my dream, how her voice was so life like and the clarity was staggering. When I awoke, I thought and dearly hoped, maybe it was all just a dream and my friend was still alive. But reality quickly set in. I soon found out that her partner had been detained for Judy's suspected murder.

To think my dear friend had died in the sanctity of her precious home, her place of refuge, where she should have been safe and protected. I felt sick at the mere thought of the fear she must have felt, what she must have gone through in her last few breaths of life. I knew she would never have really suspected or thought for a moment it would ever end like this. She had certainly never let on to me that she ever felt in danger in her own home. In my dream, which I had for three consecutive nights, I knew she was somehow trying to let me know what her final moments were like.

I was broken to think that she had suffered in the hands of a person she should have trusted. She was a little thing and had no chance of defending herself. I was angry, sad, shocked and grieving for a wonderful woman who had her life and future, her hopes and dreams snatched from her. I guess my one regret with Judy was not 'seeing the signs' of a woman who was being abused. The signs were there when I looked back, but I failed Judy by not picking up on them and helping her get away from the awful situation she was in.

She was living with domestic violence but would turn up to work every day with a smile and focus on her work. I spent many hours working alongside Judy as she was working mostly full-time, yet I feel to this day somewhat negligent in not detecting any signs that things were not right at home for her. If by speaking about this now and just one person who reads this, knows of someone, or recognizes that they are in a situation where they are abused, whether it be financial, emotional, physical, sexual or verbal they need to seek help, professional help. Speak to someone, call someone, whatever it takes for you to safely extract yourself (or loved ones) away from that situation is the most important thing for you to do.

So much domestic violence occurs yet it is a silent scourge. It goes on behind closed doors and the perpetrators of domestic violence are sadly often protected by their victims themselves. Often the victims defend the people who abuse them, as they are 'family' and the victims often feel that they themselves are the ones to blame, that they somehow 'deserve' this and would be 'nothing' without the person who is abusing them. They fear leaving that person as the perpetrators often 'threaten' them if they speak of it or make them feel they won't be able to survive without them! Victims feel this way as they are often 'put down' verbally by abusers. Abusers can control money, sex and increase the dependency of their target on them so they feel they would have nothing to start over again on their own. We have all had domestic violence touch our lives, either through someone we know, or personally.

We need to look out for each other. Reach out if you believe someone you know is in this situation, so they can feel safe to open up and speak out and seek the appropriate help they need.

This chapter is here to honor a wonderful nurse whom I will never forget. Judy, you were a wonderful friend and human being whose loss will always be felt deeply by all those who knew and loved you.

"It's what people don't say that speaks volumes."

CHAPTER 18

Nurse Call

I was called into nursing as a young child, I am now a grandmother. I have never suffered from boredom in my nursing career. Every day I have thrived in my job. It is diverse. I have the opportunity every single day to make a difference to a person in need.

If becoming a nurse is your dream, no matter what your age, you can achieve this dream and not only achieve it but excel in this wonderful profession. The desire to achieve this must come from deep within you and you must want it.

I could never have imagined how fulfilled I am nursing. Every day I wake up, keen to get to work and make a difference. To bring a smile to someone's face, to ease pain in someone who is suffering. It's the best feeling ever.

I often think what changes will occur in nursing over the next 38 years. Nursing will continue to change and develop dramatically, I am sure. Nurses will not and cannot ever be replaced by robots or computers because nurses offer a patient the humour, touch and comfort to meet their patients' needs and support their clients in a way that cannot be duplicated by any other profession. Nurses are unique in that way. Nurses have many different personalities; each has different things to bring to their nursing profession.

I have had students who struggle with certain things. I teach them how to turn this area of weakness into a strength by recognizing it and then working hard using strategies to face it and overcome that weakness. With practice, guidance and determination, I have watched these students become more confident and the quality they thought was a weakness is now a strength in their nursing practice. None of us is perfect but by facing our imperfections and working hard on them, they can become a strength and will no longer hold us back.

I will be a nurse until the day I die and just maybe you may hear talk of a 'white nurse' who walks the passageways and wards of a hospital you work in. Do not fear coming across that nurse during your night shift as it's quite likely he or she could be a welcome and unexpected helper in your busy shift. Smile and be grateful for the comfort she gives to the patients in your care. Be on the lookout for signs of her visits, such as a certain peaceful or contented look on a patient who otherwise is often grimacing in pain or wracked with stress or grief.

If you receive a 'Nurse Call' that prompts you to consider choosing nursing as your career, don't ignore it … most likely it can't be ignored. It will draw you like a moth to a light. Then you will find a world of wonder and an insatiable desire to learn more and more about this world and will grow with this knowledge to become a dedicated, compassionate nurse.

Spread your wings and fly, as your career will take you to places and people you never imagined you would discover.

You will soar with each new opportunity and experience you encounter. You will be rich with these experiences … you will be glad you answered your 'Nurse Call'.

ABOUT THE AUTHOR

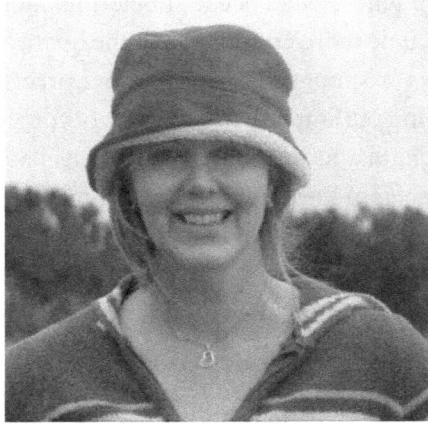

Penelope Frances wrote this book from reflections of her most poignant memories in her life that moulded her into the person she is today.

"Nurse Call" reflects on her earliest upbringing where animals were her world, as she nurtured and befriended them, to her current day student nurse facilitator role where she nurtures and teaches her precious student nurses to go out and make a positive difference every single day.

To find out more checkout her Website:
nursecallstoree.com

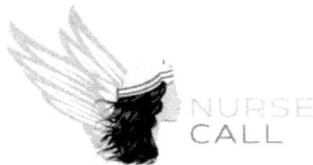

www.ingramcontent.com/pod-product-compliance
Lightning Source LLC
LaVergne TN
LVHW021541080426
835509LV00019B/2775